ACCSAP 9 VERSION

Adult Clinical Cardiology Self-Assessment Program

Book 6

Pericardial, Congenital, and Vascular Diseases

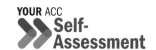

YOUR ACC
Self-Assessment

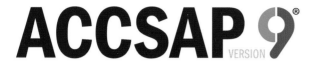

Adult Clinical Cardiology Self-Assessment Program

Book 6
Pericardial Disease

PERICARDIAL DISEASE

Editor:

James C. Fang, MD, FACC
Consultant Fees/Honoraria: Accorda; Data Safety Monitoring Board: Actelion, Cardiocell, NIH.

Pericardial Diseases   5
Barry Borlaug, MD, FACC

Pericardial Diseases

Introduction

In contrast to other areas in cardiovascular disease, there is less trial-based evidence upon which to base treatment recommendations for pericardial disease, although several recent studies have shed new light on the treatment, and guidelines from the European Society of Cardiology have been published.[1]

The pericardium is a rigid, avascular fibrous sac composed of a visceral layer adjacent to the epicardium, and a slightly thicker and richly innervated parietal layer.[2] The visceral and parietal pericardia are separated by a potential space that normally contains a small amount of lubricating fluid. The pericardium probably functions teleologically as a barrier limiting the spread of infection. The pericardium dilates with chronic cardiac enlargement (e.g., in heart failure), and may significantly contribute to the increases in intracardiac pressures observed during acute cardiac dilation, especially involving the thinner-walled right heart, as in right ventricular (RV) infarction, pulmonary embolism or subacute mitral insufficiency, or with acute increase in pericardial contents, as in cardiac tamponade.[2,3]

Pericarditis

Acute pericarditis is a relatively common source of chest pain that may be confused with coronary ischemia.[4] The vast majority (>80-90%) of cases are the result of viral infection or idiopathic pericarditis, although a large number of other causes have been described (*Table 1*).[4,5] Because the majority of cases are idiopathic, aggressive evaluation for etiology is usually deferred, but if clues from the history suggest mycobacterial, purulent, neoplastic, or collagen-vascular disease, more aggressive evaluation should be considered.[6]

The chest pain from pericarditis is quite characteristic and readily distinguished from angina.[7] Pericarditis pain may be extraordinarily severe and is most often sharp, pleuritic, and positional, relieved when

Barry Borlaug, MD, FACC
Consultant Fees/Honoraria: Amgen, GlaxoSmithKline, Merck; Pharmaceuticals: Aires Pharmaceuticals, AstraZeneca; Research/Research Grants: Medtronic.

Learner Objectives

Upon completion of this module, the reader will be able to:

1. Recognize how to diagnose, evaluate, and treat patients with acute pericarditis.
2. Discuss the pathophysiology of cardiac tamponade and relate this to physical findings and hemodynamic effects of pericardiocentesis.
3. Identify the causes of constrictive pericarditis and discuss how examination, imaging techniques, and hemodynamic assessment are optimally used to diagnose constriction.

- ○ Idiopathic

- ○ Infectious (viral, mycobacterial, fungal, purulent)

- ○ Autoimmune disease

- ○ Postcardiotomy syndrome (cardiac surgery, trauma)

- ○ Acute myocardial infarction (acute, delayed)

- ○ Neoplastic disease

- ○ Uremia

Table 1
Etiologies of Acute Pericarditis

Diagnostic Test	Finding in Pericarditis
Physical Exam	Pericardial rub
Electrocardiogram	Diffuse ST elevation and PR-segment changes
Echocardiogram	Pericardial effusion with or without tamponade
Chest X-ray	Usually normal; may see cardiomegaly "water bottle" heart shadow, pleural effusions
Blood Tests	Inflammatory markers (ESR, CRP, white blood count)
	Markers of myocardial necrosis (troponin, CK-MB)

Table 2

Routine Evaluation for Acute Pericarditis

CK-MB = creatine kinase-myocardial band;
CRP = C-reactive protein;
ESR = erythrocyte sedimentation rate.

the patient leans forward and made worse in the supine position. The pain often radiates to the trapezius ridge and may be associated with a low-grade fever or other antecedent symptoms of viral infection. Physical exam often reveals a high-pitched, scratchy pericardial rub that may contain one to three components.

Several evaluations are mandatory in the diagnostic workup for all patients presenting with possible pericarditis (*Table 2*).[1] Electrocardiography (ECG) characteristically shows diffuse ST-segment elevation and PR-segment depression early in the course of pericarditis, with the exception being lead aVR, where PR elevation is often present.[4] In later stages, there is normalization of ST-segment elevation, followed by T-wave inversions and then normalization. The simultaneous presence of both ST elevation and T-wave inversion is not seen in pericarditis and should trigger further evaluation for coronary ischemia.

Inflammatory markers such as the erythrocyte sedimentation rate and C-reactive protein may be elevated. Failure to rapidly normalize these markers with treatment predicts increased risk for recurrence.[8] Troponin may be very mildly elevated in 35-50% of patients with pericarditis because of epicardial inflammation, usually associated with normal creatine kinase-myocardial band (CK-MB).[4] When troponin values are higher and wall motion abnormalities are detected, the diagnosis of myopericarditis should be considered in addition to myocardial ischemia. Elevation in troponin levels does not carry adverse prognostic implications in the setting of myocarditis as recovery rates are generally excellent.[9]

Chest radiography may reveal pleural disease, cardiomegaly, or even the classic "water bottle" heart when a large effusion is present, though it is most often normal in acute pericarditis. Echocardiography is essential and may range from normal to small effusion with frank tamponade physiology (as noted in the following section on *Cardiac Tamponade*).

Recent guidelines suggest that the diagnosis of pericarditis requires two or more of the following: typical chest pain, ECG abnormalities, pericardial rub, and/or pericardial effusion. The presence of elevated inflammatory markers is supportive but not necessary.

Acute pericarditis as a result of viral or idiopathic disease usually responds to treatment with aspirin or nonsteroidal anti-inflammatory drugs (NSAIDs).[1,4,5,7] Options include high-dose ibuprofen (e.g., 300-800 mg every 6-8 hours), aspirin (e.g., 650 mg qid), or indomethacin (e.g., 50 mg tid) for at least 1-2 weeks. Aspirin is favored in postmyocardial infarction pericarditis, and NSAIDs (particularly indomethacin) should be avoided in these patients.[4]

Colchicine improves clinical response and has been shown in trials to reduce the risk of recurrence of pericarditis; as such, it is now recommended in addition to NSAIDs at a dose of 0.6 mg qd for patients <70 kg and 0.6 mg bid for ≥70 kg.[10,11,12] Colchicine recently has been shown to be effective to reduce incidence of the postpericardiotomy syndrome in patients undergoing cardiac surgery.[13] Corticosteroids are effective for pericarditis, but are associated with an increased risk of recurrence, and for this reason, they should be avoided if possible.[14,15]

Pericarditis as a result of specific diseases (*Table 1*) should be treated according to the primary disorder (e.g., dialysis for uremia, antibiotics, and drainage for purulent pericarditis). Many authorities recommend routine hospitalization for patients with pericarditis for initial evaluation, as noted earlier,[7] whereas other groups reserve inpatient evaluation for patients with only high-risk markers (e.g., temperature >38°C, subacute onset, tamponade or large effusion, or lack of response to aspirin or NSAIDs).[16]

Chronic or recurrent pericarditis can be managed in much the same way as acute disease, except that co-administering colchicine is recommended for even longer durations.[1] Steroid-sparing agents such as azathioprine, intravenous immunoglobulin, or anakinra have been used anecdotally in chronic or relapsing pericarditis.[1] In rare circumstances, intrapericardial injection or even pericardiectomy can be considered.

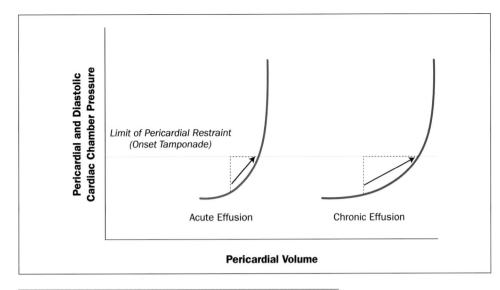

Figure 1

Pericardial Pressure-Volume Relationships

In the normal pericardium (left curve), accumulation of a small amount of pericardial fluid increases pericardial pressure to the point where the pericardium restrains cardiac filling, leading to tamponade physiology. With slowly developing, chronic effusions, the pericardium dilates (right curve), allowing accumulation of a much larger volume of fluid before tamponade physiology develops.

Key Points

- Acute pericarditis may be confused with other causes of chest pain such as coronary ischemia, aortic dissection, or pulmonary embolism. It usually can be distinguished based on the characteristics of pain, physical examination, and typical ECG changes.

- Acute pericarditis usually responds rapidly to anti-inflammatory therapy, including NSAIDs and aspirin. Colchicine improves clinical response and reduces recurrence and should be added to NSAID therapy. Corticosteroids are effective, but should be avoided because of increased risk for recurrence.

Cardiac Tamponade

Tamponade occurs when an effusion develops that is sufficient to increase total pericardial volume (i.e., heart plus effusion) from the compliant portion of the pericardial pressure-volume relationship to the steep portion (*Figure 1*).[17,18] In chronic, slowly developing effusions (e.g., neoplastic), there is pericardial remodeling and dilation, allowing a relatively large effusion to exist with no impairment in diastolic filling.

In contrast, an acute development of even a small-volume effusion, for example during a cardiac intervention, can produce cardiogenic shock and death without prompt intervention because there has not been adequate time for the pericardium to dilate (*Figure 1*). Cardiac tamponade is a correctable and life-threatening cause of cardiogenic shock that always must be considered in the patient with pulseless electrical activity.[7]

In tamponade, there is equalization of diastolic pressures in the right and left heart chambers, as they share the same effective compliance of the pericardium.[19] Ventricular and atrial filling dynamics throughout the cardiac cycle

essentially become a zero-sum game—for any increase in ventricular volume, there is a corresponding decrease in atrial volume; conversely, when right-sided filling volume increases (as during inspiration), there is a matched drop in left-sided volume.[19,20] This latter phenomenon, termed "ventricular interdependence," produces the exaggerated drop in systolic blood pressure (>10 mm Hg) during inspiration, known as "pulsus paradoxus."[21]

The presence of pulsus paradoxus increases the odds of cardiac tamponade more than threefold, while its absence makes tamponade very unlikely.[22] Patients with tamponade usually appear in distress, with complaints of dyspnea, fatigue, air hunger, altered mentation, or chest pain.[17] Jugular distention is typically present, and characteristic loss of the Y descent is noted, as early diastolic filling is impaired.[23] Tachycardia is the rule and is related to drop in stroke volume from impairment in diastolic ventricular filling. Blood pressure may be normal as reflex sympathetic activation increases arterial resistance and heart rate to maintain perfusion. A paradoxical pulse should be assessed in all patients; this can be palpable during inspiration when significant tamponade is present, or may be auscultated by slowly deflating a blood pressure cuff while observing the timing of the first Korotkoff sound relative to respiration.

The paradoxical pulse may be difficult to appreciate in patients with hypotension or tachypnea, or it may be absent if there is an atrial septal defect, reduced left ventricular (LV) compliance, or aortic insufficiency.[17,24] Heart sounds may be muffled, and a rub may be noted if the effusion is a result of an inflammatory process. Kussmaul's sign (inspiratory increase in jugular venous pressure) is usually absent unless constrictive, tricuspid, or myocardial disease is also present.

It should be emphasized that cardiac tamponade is a *clinical* diagnosis that is not made by any one single test.[17] Echocardiography is the single most useful noninvasive test used to help determine the hemodynamic significance of an effusion. Tamponade usually is associated with circumferential effusions, often with collapse of the thin-walled right atrium and RV during diastole.[7] Enhanced ventricular interdependence is detected by a significant drop in transmitral inflow by pulse-wave Doppler during inspiration.[25] This is mirrored by an increase in transtricuspid flow velocities. Systemic venous hypertension is detected by caval distention and failure to normally collapse during inspiration.

ECG reveals sinus tachycardia with low voltage.[17] There also may be variation in the amplitude of the QRS complex with every other beat (electrical alternans), and while this finding is not common, it is highly specific for cardiac tamponade. Very large effusions (>200 ml) produce cardiomegaly on chest radiography, but heart size is normal with smaller effusions.[17]

Guidelines on the evaluation, triage, and management for tamponade were published recently.[26] Intravenous fluids may provide some support while awaiting definitive therapy, with an increase in cardiac output observed in about one-half of patients.[27] Inotropes and pressors are usually of little value because intrinsic catecholamine levels are very high and the pathophysiologic mechanism is a diastolic process, not systolic or vascular.[7] Initiating positive pressure ventilation in a patient with tamponade can be catastrophic, as the increase in intrathoracic pressure further limits chamber filling.[28] The only definitive treatment for tamponade is pericardiocentesis. This can be performed surgically in the catheterization laboratory or, more commonly today, using echocardiographic guidance at the bedside.[28] Pigtail catheters are usually left in place for at least 24 hours.

A large pericardial effusion causing tamponade in the absence of obvious causes (e.g., inflammatory pericarditis, cardiac surgery) should prompt further evaluation for malignancy, and aspirated fluid should be sent for cytology, along with other studies. One study has found that one-third of large (>20 mm) pericardial effusions will eventually progress to tamponade,[29] but the management of these chronic large effusions without tamponade remains controversial.[6]

Key Points

- Cardiac tamponade is a life-threatening cause of cardiogenic shock that can develop acutely or chronically, and should be suspected in a patient with tachycardia, jugular distention, or pulseless electrical activity.

- Tamponade is a clinical diagnosis with key findings including paradoxical pulse on exam and characteristic echocardiographic abnormalities including right heart collapse and significant respiratory variation in LV filling on echocardiography. Intravenous fluids may improve cardiac output, but pericardiocentesis is the only definitive therapy.

Constrictive Pericarditis

Constrictive pericarditis develops in response to subacute or chronic inflammation with scarring, thickening, and fibrosis of the pericardium.[1,30] There are multiple causes, but by far the most common in the developed world include radiation, idiopathic, and prior cardiac surgery.[31] In constriction, a reduction in pericardial space because of fibrosis reduces all cardiac chamber volumes, producing competition for diastolic filling, equalization of diastolic pressures, and enhanced ventricular interdependence, similar to what is seen in cardiac tamponade.

Patients with constriction typically present with symptoms of fatigue and exertional dyspnea.[1] There also may be symptoms related to abdominal distention, such as anorexia and early satiety. There is usually dramatic evidence of systemic venous congestion, with peripheral edema, ascites, and pulsatile hepatomegaly. Lung fields are generally clear, but pleural effusion may be noted. Jugular venous distention is the rule, but because this may not always be appreciated on examination, it is not uncommon for such patients to have undergone extensive workup for hepatobiliary disease prior to presenting to a cardiologist. The jugular pulsations reveal prominent X and Y descents, especially during inspiration, where jugular pressure increases (Kussmaul's sign; *Figure 2*). Cardiac auscultation may reveal a high-pitched early diastolic sound (pericardial knock) that corresponds to the rapid deceleration of ventricular inflow. When constriction is severe, cardiac output is low, leading to vasoconstriction to maintain adequate blood pressure, detectable on examination by cool extremities.

Pericardial constriction may be confused with restrictive cardiomyopathy or garden variety heart failure with preserved ejection fraction ("diastolic" heart failure). Pericardial calcification and/or thickening noted on plain films, chest computed tomography (CT), or magnetic resonance imaging (MRI) make constriction the more likely diagnosis, although 18% of patients with constriction may have normal pericardial thickness.[32]

Doppler echocardiography is extremely useful to distinguish constrictive and restrictive disease, with constriction showing significant respiratory variation in mitral inflow (>25% drop during inspiration) and hepatic vein flow reversal during expiration.[33] In constriction, a septal "bounce" or "notch" may be detected on two-dimensional imaging or M-mode, respectively, corresponding to the timing of the pericardial knock on exam, although this must be distinguished from other septal motion abnormalities related to pacing or left bundle branch block. Echocardiographic criteria to distinguish pericardial constriction from myocardial diseases have been published recently.[34]

Tissue Doppler echocardiography has emerged as a useful discriminative tool in the evaluation—patients with restrictive disease typically have low early diastolic tissue velocities (E'), whereas E' are normal or elevated in

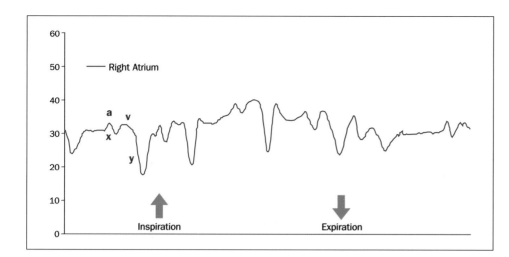

Figure 2

Right Atrial Pressure Tracing in a Patient With Constrictive Pericarditis

The Y descent is prominent, and rather than the normal fall in mean pressure during inspiration, there is an increase noted. This is referred to as a positive Kussmaul's sign and is frequently seen in pericardial and right heart disease.

pericardial constriction, particularly at the mitral annular septum.[35-37] Biatrial enlargement tends to be more severe in myocardial disease, but may be seen to a lesser extent in constriction. Caval plethora with lack of inspiratory collapse reflects right atrial hypertension and is common to both constriction and restriction. B-type natriuretic peptide levels, which vary directly with ventricular wall stress, are less elevated in constriction compared with heart failure or restriction,[38] probably because the pericardial constraining effect limits ventricular stretch.

Constriction usually can be distinguished from restrictive disease based on examination and careful imaging assessment,[33] but when uncertainty persists, invasive hemodynamic assessment is required. Catheterization remains the "gold standard" and requires simultaneous assessment of right- and left-sided intracardiac pressures with and without dynamic respiratory maneuvers.[39,40] A normal cardiac output in the setting of normal right atrial pressure makes clinically relevant constriction very unlikely. Traditional findings favoring constriction over restrictive disease include equalization of RV and LV end-diastolic pressures, absence of pulmonary hypertension, "dip and plateau" diastolic ventricular waveforms in both ventricles, high ratio of RV diastolic pressure to systolic pressure (greater than one-third), and positive Kussmaul's sign.[23] However, recent studies have shown that these findings often are seen in restrictive disease or causes of heart failure and, thus, lack specificity.[40]

Dynamic respiratory maneuvers distinguish constriction from restriction with much greater sensitivity and specificity (>90%).[40] These maneuvers rely on two characteristic pathophysiologic observations in constriction: 1) enhanced ventricular interdependence, and 2) dissociation between intrathoracic and intracardiac pressures. The latter is produced by an "insulating" effect of the thickened, fibrotic pericardium, such that the negative intrathoracic pressure generated during deep inspiration is not fully transmitted to the LV, but still reduces pressure in extracardiac structures including the pulmonary veins.

As a result, the gradient favoring transfer of blood from pulmonary veins to the left atrium and LV is reduced. This can be identified by the reduction in transmitral E-wave velocity on echocardiography,[33] or a drop in the diastolic gradient between pulmonary wedge pressure and LV diastolic pressure by catheterization (*Figure 3*).[40] Because of enhanced ventricular interdependence in constriction, the RV takes advantage of this transient left-sided underfilling during inspiration: the septum bows from right to left, and RV preload increases. As a result, LV systolic pressure decreases while RV pressure increases in constriction (discordance; *Figure 4*). In restriction, pressure changes in the two ventricles occur in phase (concordance).

Severe tricuspid insufficiency with right heart failure may produce hemodynamics that are very similar to constriction, with equalization of diastolic pressures, ventricular "dip and plateau," and some interdependence, but the latter is usually mild, and the RV diastolic pressure frequently exceeds the LV during deep inspiration, helping to discern the two entities. In some patients with apparent cardiac tamponade taken for pericardiocentesis, cardiac filling pressures remain elevated despite drainage of the pericardial fluid and normalization of pericardial pressure. This is a result of coexisting constriction and inflammation of the visceral pericardium. This variant, which probably represents a transition from acute inflammatory pericarditis to constrictive disease, is termed "effusive-constrictive pericarditis."[41]

The treatment of constrictive pericarditis is surgical pericardiectomy.[30,31] In some cases, particularly when there is more evidence for ongoing pericardial inflammation (e.g., elevated inflammatory markers, hyper-enhancement by MRI), a course of anti-inflammatory therapy with NSAIDs, colchicine, or corticosteroids can effectively treat the inflammatory process causing constriction, without the need for surgery.[42] Patients with constriction as a result of prior radiation in general fair much more poorly with pericardiectomy compared with other causes, likely because there is often coexisting myocardial, valvular, and coronary disease related to prior radiation exposure.[31]

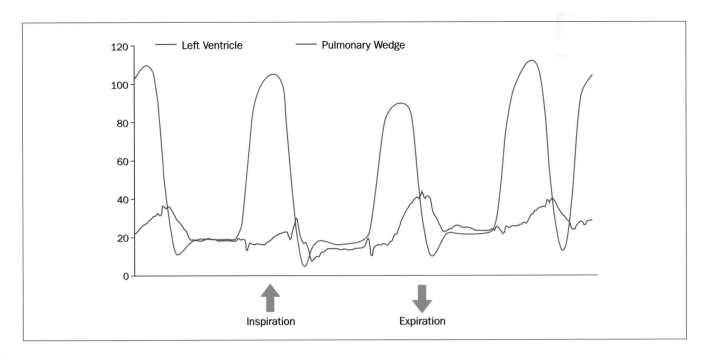

Figure 3

LV and Pulmonary Wedge Pressure Tracings in Constriction

Normally left ventricular (LV) diastolic and wedge pressures move in synchrony during respiration, such that the diastolic gradient from wedge to LV remains constant. In constriction, negative intrathoracic pressure "pulls" wedge pressure below LV diastolic, with the converse occurring during expiration. This is termed "intrathoracic-intracardiac dissociation" and is a sensitive and specific sign of constrictive pericarditis.

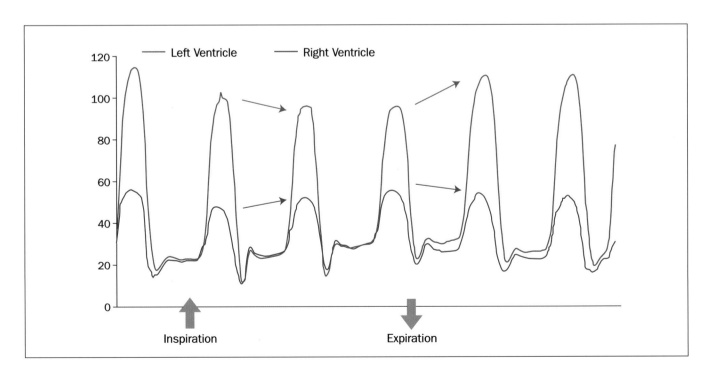

Figure 4

LV and RV Pressure Tracings During Deep Breathing in Constrictive Pericarditis

As a result of enhanced ventricular interdependence, the systolic area under the right ventricular (RV) pressure tracing increases during inspiration while the left ventricular (LV) systolic area decreases (arrows). The opposite occurs during expiration.

Key Points

- Echocardiography is often diagnostic of constriction. Key findings include abnormal septal motion, diastolic tissue Doppler velocities that are higher in the septum than the lateral wall, abnormal septal motion, and increased respiratory variation in the mitral inflow velocities.

- Constrictive pericarditis is an important cause of right-sided heart failure that should be suspected when marked systemic venous congestion is present and past history suggests possible causes such as prior chest radiation, cardiothoracic surgery, or episodes of recurrent pericarditis.

- Constrictive pericarditis can be diagnosed frequently by history, physical examination, and imaging, but catheterization remains the "gold standard." Catheterization findings rely on equalization of filling pressures, enhanced ventricular interdependence, and intrathoracic-interventricular dissociation. The diagnosis of constriction should be aggressively pursued because it is a reversible cause of heart failure symptoms.

Future Directions

The pathophysiology causing recurrent pericarditis remains unclear. In the future, more detailed evaluation for specific etiologies causing recurrent acute episodes may allow for more efficacious and focused treatments directed at the underlying cause, including infections and autoimmune syndromes. Constrictive pericarditis can be one of the more gratifying cardiovascular diseases to treat, with complete "cure" for heart failure symptoms with pericardiectomy, but the surgery remains high risk in comparison with other cardiovascular surgeries, and many patients continue to complain of symptoms after pericardial resection.

Future research should seek to identify and stratify the patients most or least likely to derive benefit and should explore how to prevent or mitigate the fibrotic process causing pericardial constriction in patients earlier on in the disease course. Pericardial disease has emerged from a field of "expert opinion" to the beginnings of an evidence base, but more trial data are required. The field will benefit greatly from a new set of diagnostic and management guidelines.

References

1. Adler Y, Charron P, Imazio M, et al. 2015 ESC guidelines for the diagnosis and management of pericardial diseases: the Task Force for the Diagnosis and Management of Pericardial Diseases of the European Society of Cardiology (ESC) endorsed by: the European Association for Cardio-Thoracic Surgery (EACTS). Eur Heart J 2015;36:2921-64.

2. Watkins MW, LeWinter MM. Physiologic role of the normal pericardium. Annu Rev Med 1993;44:171-80.

3. Freeman GL, LeWinter MM. Pericardial adaptations during chronic cardiac dilation in dogs. Circ Res 1984;54:294-300.

4. Lange RA, Hillis LD. Clinical practice. Acute pericarditis. N Engl J Med 2004;351:2195-202.

5. Spodick DH. Acute pericarditis: current concepts and practice. JAMA 2003;289:1150-3.

6. Imazio M, Spodick DH, Brucato A, Trinchero R, Adler Y. Controversial issues in the management of pericardial diseases. Circulation 2010;121:916-28.

7. Little WC, Freeman GL. Pericardial disease. Circulation 2006;113:1622-32.

8. Imazio M, Brucato A, Maestroni S, et al. Prevalence of C-reactive protein elevation and time course of normalization in acute pericarditis: implications for the diagnosis, therapy, and prognosis of pericarditis. Circulation 2011;123:1092-7.

9. Imazio M, Brucato A, Barbieri A, et al. Good prognosis for pericarditis with and without myocardial involvement: results from a multicenter, prospective cohort study. Circulation 2013;128:42-9.

10. Imazio M, Brucato A, Cemin R, et al. A randomized trial of colchicine for acute pericarditis. N Engl J Med 2013;369:1522-8.

11. Imazio M, Belli R, Brucato A, et al. Efficacy and safety of colchicine for treatment of multiple recurrences of pericarditis (CORP-2): a multicentre, double-blind, placebo-controlled, randomised trial. Lancet 2014;383:2232-7.

12. Imazio M, Bobbio M, Cecchi E, et al. Colchicine in addition to conventional therapy for acute pericarditis: results of the COlchicine for acute PEricarditis (COPE) trial. Circulation 2005;112:2012-6.

13. Imazio M, Brucato A, Ferrazzi P, et al., on behalf of the COPPS-2 Investigators. Colchicine for prevention of postpericardiotomy syndrome and postoperative atrial fibrillation: the COPPS-2 randomized clinical trial. JAMA 2014;312:1016-23.

14. Imazio M, Brucato A, Cumetti D, et al. Corticosteroids for recurrent pericarditis: high versus low doses: a nonrandomized observation. Circulation 2008;118:667-71.

15. Imazio M, Cecchi E, Demichelis B, et al. Indicators of poor prognosis of acute pericarditis. Circulation 2007;115:2739-44.

16. Imazio M, Demichelis B, Parrini I, et al. Day-hospital treatment of acute pericarditis: a management program for outpatient therapy. J Am Coll Cardiol 2004;43:1042-6.

17. Spodick DH. Acute cardiac tamponade. N Engl J Med 2003;349:684-90.

18. Reddy PS, Curtiss EI, O'Toole JD, Shaver JA. Cardiac tamponade: hemodynamic observations in man. Circulation 1978;58:265-72.

19. Shabetai R. Pericardial effusion: haemodynamic spectrum. Heart 2004;90:255-6.

20. Hess OM, Bhargava V, Ross J Jr, Shabetai R. The role of the pericardium in interactions between the cardiac chambers. Am Heart J 1983;106:1377-83.

21. Shabetai R, Fowler NO, Fenton JC, Masangkay M. Pulsus paradoxus. J Clin Invest 1965;44:1882-98.

22. Curtiss EI, Reddy PS, Uretsky BF, Cecchetti AA. Pulsus paradoxus: definition and relation to the severity of cardiac tamponade. Am Heart J 1988;115:391-8.

23. Shabetai R, Fowler NO, Guntheroth WG. The hemodynamics of cardiac tamponade and constrictive pericarditis. Am J Cardiol 1970;26:480-9.

24. Hoit BD, Gabel M, Fowler NO. Cardiac tamponade in left ventricular dysfunction. Circulation 1990;82:1370-6.

25. Gonzalez MS, Basnight MA, Appleton CP. Experimental pericardial effusion: relation of abnormal respiratory variation in mitral flow velocity to hemodynamics and diastolic right heart collapse. J Am Coll Cardiol 1991;17:239-48.

26. Ristic AD, Imazio M, Adler Y, et al. Triage strategy for urgent management of cardiac tamponade: a position statement of the European Society of Cardiology Working Group on Myocardial and Pericardial Diseases. Eur Heart J 2014; 35:2279-84.

27. Sagristà-Sauleda J, Angel J, Sambola A, Permanyer-Miralda G. Hemodynamic effects of volume expansion in patients with cardiac tamponade. Circulation 2008;117:1545-9.

28. Tsang TS, Barnes ME, Hayes SN, et al. Clinical and echocardiographic characteristics of significant pericardial effusions following cardiothoracic surgery and outcomes of echo-guided pericardiocentesis for management: Mayo Clinic experience, 1979-1998. Chest 1999;116:322-31.

29. Sagristà-Sauleda J, Angel J, Permanyer-Miralda G, Soler-Soler J. Long-term follow-up of idiopathic chronic pericardial effusion. N Engl J Med 1999;341:2054-9.

30. Hoit BD. Management of effusive and constrictive pericardial heart disease. Circulation 2002;105:2939-42.

31. Ling LH, Oh JK, Schaff HV, et al. Constrictive pericarditis in the modern era: evolving clinical spectrum and impact on outcome after pericardiectomy. Circulation 1999;100:1380-6.

32. Talreja DR, Edwards WD, Danielson GK, et al. Constrictive pericarditis in 26 patients with histologically normal pericardial thickness. Circulation 2003;108:1852-7.

33. Oh JK, Hatle LK, Seward JB, et al. Diagnostic role of Doppler echocardiography in constrictive pericarditis. J Am Coll Cardiol 1994;23:154-62.

34. Welch TD, Ling LH, Espinosa RE, et al. Echocardiographic diagnosis of constrictive pericarditis: Mayo Clinic criteria. Circ Cardiovasc Imaging 2014; 7:526-34.

35. Rajagopalan N, Garcia MJ, Rodriguez L, et al. Comparison of new Doppler echocardiographic methods to differentiate constrictive pericardial heart disease and restrictive cardiomyopathy. Am J Cardiol 2001;87:86-94.

36. Garcia MJ, Rodriguez L, Ares M, Griffin BP, Thomas JD, Klein AL. Differentiation of constrictive pericarditis from restrictive cardiomyopathy: assessment of left ventricular diastolic velocities in longitudinal axis by Doppler tissue imaging. J Am Coll Cardiol 1996;27:108-14.

37. Ha JW, Ommen SR, Tajik AJ, et al. Differentiation of constrictive pericarditis from restrictive cardiomyopathy using mitral annular velocity by tissue Doppler echocardiography. Am J Cardiol 2004;94:316-9.

38. Babuin L, Alegria JR, Oh JK, Nishimura RA, Jaffe AS. Brain natriuretic peptide levels in constrictive pericarditis and restrictive cardiomyopathy. J Am Coll Cardiol 2006;47:1489-91.

39. Talreja DR, Nishimura RA, Oh JK, Holmes DR. Constrictive pericarditis in the modern era: novel criteria for diagnosis in the cardiac catheterization laboratory. J Am Coll Cardiol 2008;51:315-9.

40. Hurrell DG, Nishimura RA, Higano ST, et al. Value of dynamic respiratory changes in left and right ventricular pressures for the diagnosis of constrictive pericarditis. Circulation 1996;93:2007-13.

41. Sagristà-Sauleda J, Angel J, Sánchez A, Permanyer-Miralda G, Soler-Soler J. Effusive-constrictive pericarditis. N Engl J Med 2004;350:469-75.

42. Haley JH, Tajik AJ, Danielson GK, Schaff HV, Mulvagh SL, Oh JK. Transient constrictive pericarditis: causes and natural history. J Am Coll Cardiol 2004;43:271-5.

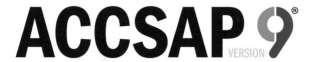

Adult Clinical Cardiology Self-Assessment Program

Book 6
Congenital Heart Disease

CONGENITAL HEART DISEASE

Editor:

Thomas M. Bashore, MD, FACC
This author has nothing to disclose.

Congenital Heart Disease
General Considerations

Introduction

Today, there are an estimated 1.25 million adults living with congenital heart disease (CHD) in the United States.[1] About 85% of patients born with CHD now live to adulthood. This 85% is made up of 46% with simple lesions (atrial septal defects [ASDs], pulmonary valve stenosis, etc.), 38% with moderately complex anatomy (tetralogy of Fallot [TOF], etc.), and 16% with great complexity (D-transposition of the great arteries [D-TGA], tricuspid or pulmonary atresia, etc.).[2]

Essentially, all patients with great complexity and most with moderate complexity will have had surgical procedures during childhood in order to survive until adulthood. Many with simple lesions will also have had interventions. Thus, the adult population is a group wherein both the native and the reconstructed anatomy play a role in the clinical status. Improved surgical outcomes have resulted in many children reaching adulthood (*Figure 1*).[3] There are now more adults living with CHD than there are children living with it (*Figure 2*).[4]

The 2008 American College of Cardiology/American Heart Association (ACC/AHA) 2008 Guidelines for the Management of Adults With Congenital Heart Disease[2] are currently undergoing revision; new guidelines will be available in 2016. In 2010, guidelines on the management of adults with CHD were published by the Canadian

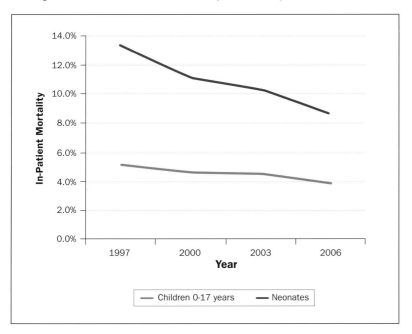

Figure 1
Improved Cardiac Surgical Outcomes in Children With Congenital Heart Disease

Reproduced with permission from Kaltman JR, Andropoulos DB, Checchia PA, et al. Report of the Pediatric Heart Network and National Heart, Lung, and Blood Institute Working Group on the Perioperative Management of Congenital Heart Disease. Circulation 2010;121:2766-72.

Thomas M. Bashore, MD, FACC
This author has nothing to disclose.

Learner Objectives

Upon completion of this module, the reader will be able to:
1. Recognize the prevalence of congenital heart disease (CHD) in adults.
2. Identify the various genetic syndromes, but focus on only those that commonly are associated with CHD.
3. Recall the Fontan anatomy and physiology in order to appreciate complications that occur.
4. Interpret the impact of cardiopulmonary stress parameters on outcomes.
5. Recognize which congenital lesions are most likely to result in sudden death.
6. Describe how heart failure and hypertension treatment in adult patients with CHD differs from those without CHD.
7. Explain which arrhythmias are associated with which congenital heart defect lesions.
8. Better summarize the prognosis in patients with Eisenmenger syndrome and how to diagnose and treat the complications.
9. Identify what the guidelines recommend regarding infective endocarditis prophylaxis and preoperative risk assessment.

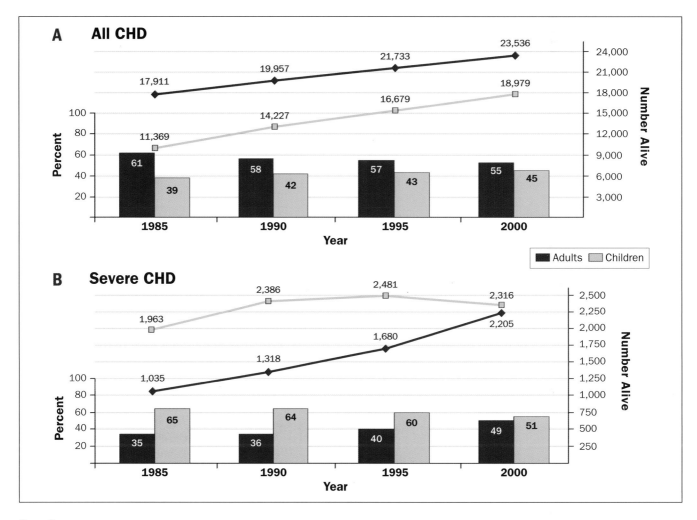

Figure 2

More Adults Now Live With Congenital Heart Disease Than Do Children

CHD = congenital heart disease.

Reproduced with permission from Marelli AJ, Mackie AS, Ionescu-Ittu R, Rahme E, Pilote L. Congenital heart disease in the general population: changing prevalence and age distribution. Circulation 2007;115:163-72.

Cardiovascular Society[5] and the European Society of Cardiology.[6] In addition, an AHA scientific statement regarding the adult CHD population was published in 2015.[1] All of these are good resources for understanding this unique and growing population of patients.

This chapter outlines common features encountered in dealing with adults with CHD, and is geared toward presenting overview knowledge rather than an in-depth discussion. Individual lesions are discussed in the other modules in this chapter.

Key Point

- There are an estimated 1.25 million adults living with CHD in the United States. 85% of those born with CHD live until adulthood. There are more adults living with CHD than children living with it.

Genetic Syndromes

There are a variety of genetic syndromes associated with patients who have CHD (*Table 1*).[7] These include chromosomal abnormalities and a variety of Mendelian syndromes. Most of these are uncommon.

The syndromes most likely to be encountered in an adult cardiology practice include Down syndrome (trisomy 21), Turner syndrome (absence or abnormality of one of the X chromosomes), and Marfan syndrome (fibrillin-1 mutation on chromosome 15q21). Children with Down syndrome typically have an atrioventricular (AV) septal defect. This defect may vary in presentation, but includes either an ASD (primum), ventricular septal defect, or both. A partial AV septal defect is present when only one of the defects is present. In complete AV septal defect, the AV valve may "float" between the upper and lower chambers. In partial AV septal defects, the five-leaflet AV valve

Table 1
Genetic Syndromes

These data are also available at *www.ncbi. nlm.nih.gov/pmc/articles/ PMC2671242*.

Reproduced with permission from Lin AE, Basson CT, Goldmuntz E, et al. Adults with genetic syndromes and cardiovascular abnormalities: clinical history and management. Genet Med 2008;10:469-94.

Chromosomal Abnormality Syndromes
○ 22q11.2 deletion: multiple phenotypes (tetralogy of Fallot, pulmonary stenosis, interrupted arch, ventricular septal defect, double outlet right ventricle, D-transposition of the great arteries, DiGeorge syndrome: CATCH-22
○ Trisomy 21: Down syndrome
○ Absence or abnormality in one of X chromosomes: Turner syndrome
○ Microdeletion on 7q and others: Williams syndrome
Mendelian Syndromes
○ Fibrillin-1 mutation: Marfan syndrome
○ TGF beta receptor disorder (TGFBR1 or TGFBR2): Loeys-Dietz syndrome
○ TBX5 gene mutation: Holt-Oram syndrome

Type	Recurrence Risk
Aortic valve septal defect	4.0%
Atrial septal defect	3.0%
Tetralogy of Fallot	3.0%
Left-sided obstructive lesions*	3.0%
Transposition of the great arteries	1.8%

* Left-sided obstructive lesions do not include the bicuspid aortic valve or its associated aortopathy.

Table 2
Risk of Transmitting Phenotype to Offspring

Reproduced with permission from Sund KL, Gawde SH, Benson DW. Adults with congenital heart disease: a genetic perspective. In: Gatzoulis MA, Webb GD, Daubeney PEF, eds. Diagnosis and Management of Adult Congenital Heart Disease. 2nd ed. Philadephia: Elsevier Saunders, 2010:16.

appears to have "clefts." Most patients (>75%) with a complete AV septal defect will have a Down's phenotype. There are a variety of 22q11.2 deletion syndromes, including the DiGeorge syndrome, which are often associated with the mnemonic CATCH-22: C = cardiac, A = abnormal facies, T = thymic aplasia and immune deficits, C = cleft palate, H = hypocalcemia/ hypoparathyroidism. The specifics of these syndromes are beyond the scope of this chapter, but can be found on the National Center for Biotechnology Information website (*www.ncbi.nlm.nih.gov/pmc/articles/PMC2671242*).

Table 2 presents the risk of transmitting certain phenotypes to progeny. Of note, the transmission of the bicuspid aortic valve and/or the associated aortopathy has been found to be much higher (up to 30%) than any of the other congenital heart defects.[8] In patients with Turner syndrome, the most common congenital abnormality is the associated aortic coarctation with a bicuspid aortic valve. In general, most congenital heart defects have about a 2-4% transmission rate to offspring. This is not the case with some of the Mendelian disorders such as Marfan syndrome, which may be autosomal dominant.

Table 3 outlines the most common phenotypes that should alert the practicing physician to the presence of underlying CHD. When these phenotypes are observed, it behooves the practicing cardiologist to seek further information to exclude an inherited cardiac abnormality.

Key Points

- The most common genetic disorders that are associated with CHD are two of the chromosomal abnormalities—trisomy 21 (Down syndrome) and the absence of an abnormality of one of the X chromosomes (Turner syndrome). The most common Mendelian congenital disorder, besides bicuspid aortic valve, is the fibrillin-1 mutation that causes Marfan syndrome.

  ○ The most common defect in Down syndrome is a complete or partial AV septal defect with abnormal "clefts" in the mitral and tricuspid valves. More than 75% of patients with a complete AV septal defect will have Down syndrome.

  ○ Other common phenotypes associated with CHD include Holt-Oram (secundum ASD) and Turner syndrome (coarctation of the aorta and a bicuspid aortic valve).

- In patients with a bicuspid aortic valve, the prevalence of either the bicuspid aortic valve and/or the aortopathy is up to 30% in first-degree relatives. Otherwise the transmission of most CHD is in the range of 1-4% to the progeny.

Down Syndrome		
	○ 60% have some congenital heart lesion.	
	○ Atrioventricular septal defect (atrial septal defects, ventricular septal defects, or both; cleft atrioventricular leaflets)	
Holt-Oram Syndrome (abnormal digits, usually thumbs; can be both upper limbs)		
	○ Secundum atrial septal defect (occasionally others)	
Noonan Sydrome (web neck, hypertelorism, low-set ears, micrognathia)		
	○ Dysplasic pulmonary valve	
Marfan Syndrome		
	○ Aortic aneurysm	
	○ Mitral valve prolapse	
	○ Aortic valve prolapse	
	○ Pulmonary artery dilatation	

Table 3
Phenotypes and Their Most Common Congenital Heart Lesions

The Glenn and Fontan Procedures

The Glenn and Fontan procedures are employed whenever a congenital anatomy requires routing blood from the systemic venous system to the pulmonary arterial system. Generally, this is related to tricuspid or pulmonary atresia, although it can be employed with other complex lesions when appropriate. Because this palliative procedure creates its own set of problems and is mentioned throughout this module, it is useful to describe the surgery at this time. *Figure 3a* outlines the Glenn procedure and *Figure 3b* outlines the Fontan procedure.

The classic or original Glenn procedure resulted in performing a cavopulmonary connection between the superior vena cava (SVC) and the disconnected right pulmonary artery (RPA). Over time, however, it was discovered that patients who only perfused the right lung via the SVC were particularly susceptible to the development of pulmonary AV malformations and cyanosis. At times these AV fistulae could become quite large. This issue was eliminated when a bidirectional Glenn procedure was performed attaching the SVC to the RPA and oversewing the pulmonary valve so that SVC blood goes to both lungs.

There are a number of ways to perform the Fontan procedure. All result in routing the inferior vena cava (IVC) blood to the lungs. The classic Fontan procedure simply attached the atrial appendage to the main PA directly, as shown in *Figure 3b*. In this example, no Glenn procedure is performed.

More recently, the procedure is generally performed by creating a tunnel from the IVC to the RPA. The insertion of the Fontan to the RPA is offset from that of an associated Glenn insertion to prevent competitive flow conflict. The main PA is oversewn and thus all SVC and IVC blood flows through both lungs without a right ventricle (RV). Because the lung will not have been accustomed to the flow, the pulmonary resistance may be high when the procedure is initially performed. The resulting backpressure in the Fontan conduit may be high as well, and most of these lateral tunnel procedures are "fenestrated" to allow for some "pop-off" flow into the right atrium (RA) to initially reduce the pressure within the conduit. Once the lungs have adapted to the new increase in flow, this fenestration is generally closed with a closure device.

Flow through the Fontan requires that the systemic venous pressure exceed the PA pressure and that active early diastolic relaxation of the systemic ventricle (usually the left ventricle [LV] is present) be normal. The hemodynamics created by the Fontan thus fails whenever there is pulmonary hypertension from any cause (pulmonary vascular disease or an elevated pulmonary venous pressure from ventricular dysfunction or AV valve regurgitation, for instance).

Arrhythmias are poorly tolerated and, unfortunately, atrial arrhythmias are common, especially intra-atrial re-entrant tachycardias. These often require antiarrhythmics and/ or atrial ablation. One option is to reduce the amount of atrial tissue available to sustain the arrhythmias by use of a MAZE procedure and/or conversion of the Fontan to

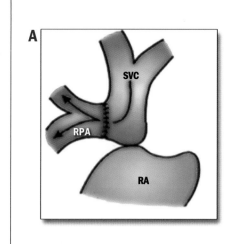 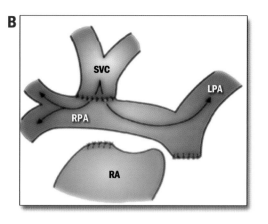

Figure 3a

The Glenn and Fontan Procedures (1 of 2)

Panel A: The classic Glenn procedure that directly connected the SVC to the RPA only. **Panel B:** The bidirectional Glenn procedure that tied off the main PA and connected the SVC in end-to-side fashion to the RPA.

RA = right atrium;
LPA = left pulmonary artery;
RPA = right pulmonary artery;
SVC = superior vena cava.

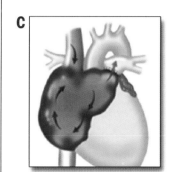 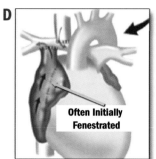 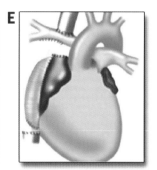

Often Initially Fenestrated

Figure 3b

The Glenn and Fontan Procedures (2 of 2)

Panel C: The classic Fontan routing blood from the right atrial appendage to the pulmonary artery. **Panel D:** The lateral tunnel Fontan through the right atrium and often initially fenestrated. **Panel E:** The extracardiac Fontan.

Reproduced with permission from Ermis PR, Morales DL. The adult Fontan patient: update for 2011. Methodist Debakey Cardiovasc J 2011;7:3-8.

an extracardiac Fontan and resection of redundant atrial tissue (*Figure 3b*).

Table 4 lists long-term complications related to the Fontan procedure. Not only is there intolerance of pulmonary hypertension and arrhythmias, the low flow state within the conduit and the atria can result in thrombus formation and an associated coagulopathy. The majority of Fontan patients are on at least aspirin (and most are on warfarin) for that reason.[9,10]

In addition, the higher pressure that occurs within the hepatic veins can eventually result in liver cirrhosis and a frighteningly high incidence of hepatocellular carcinoma.[11] All Fontan patients should thus have yearly liver function tests and alpha-fetoprotein measurements.

Finally, a peculiar loss of protein into the gut occurs when the Fontan physiology begins to fail. This protein-losing enteropathy is often a harbinger of a poor prognosis.[12] It can be detected by serial measurement of a drop in the serum albumin and diagnosed by testing the feces for the presence of the protein alpha-1 antitrypsin.

Key Points

- Cyanosis in a patient with a classic Glenn procedure may be due to the formation of pulmonary AV malformations.

- A reduction in the occurrence of atrial arrhythmias in patients with a lateral tunnel Fontan may be improved by conversion to an extracardiac Fontan.

- There is a higher than expected incidence of hepatocellular carcinoma in patients who have had a Fontan procedure.

- A poor prognostic sign in patients with a Fontan is the presence of a protein-losing enteropathy.

Exercise Intolerance

Patients with CHD often have significant limitations in their exercise tolerance, depending on their anatomy and hemodynamics. This is often objectively assessed by use of

- No toleration for pulmonary hypertension from ANY cause
- Poor toleration of atrial arrhythmias
- Coagulopathy
- Liver dysfunction and cirrhosis
- Liver cancer (hepatocellular carcinoma)
- Protein-losing enteropathy

Table 4

Long-Term Complications in Patients With the Fontan Procedure

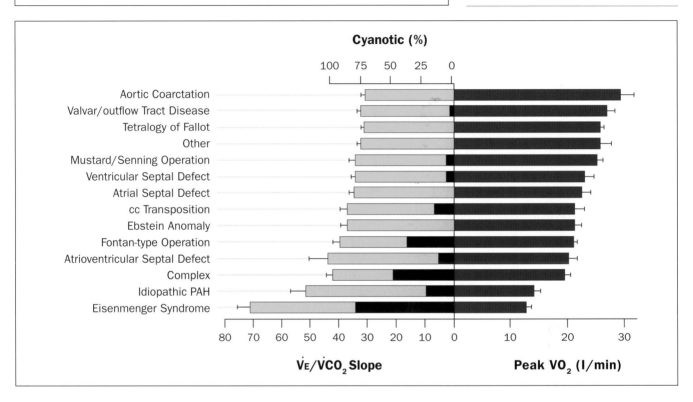

Figure 4

Exercise Intolerance in Patients With Congenital Heart Disease

The more rapid the V_E/VCO_2 slope or the lower the peak VO_2, the more the exercise limitation. The percent of patients in each group with cyanosis is shown in black.

cc = congenitally corrected; PAH = pulmonary arterial hypertension.

Reproduced with permission from Dimoulos K, Alonso-Gonzalex ET, Gatzoulis, MA. Heart failure, exercise intolerance, and physical training. In: Gatzoulis MA, Webb GD, Daubeney PEF, eds. Diagnosis and Management of Adult Congenital Heart Disease. 2nd ed. Philadephia: Elsevier Saunders, 2010:47.

cardiopulmonary exercise testing.[13] An adequate test can be defined by the peak respiratory exchange rate of ≥1.10. This is the ratio between VCO_2 and VO_2. The two most important parameters obtained from the cardiopulmonary exercise are the VO_2 max (maximal aerobic capacity) and the minute ventilation-carbon dioxide output relationship (V_E/VCO_2).

The greater the VO_2 max, the better the exercise performance. It is defined as the amount of oxygen a person takes up and delivers to the tissue at peak exercise at the point where the oxygen consumption plateaus despite increasing work rate. A level <14 L/kg/

min is considered a threshold value to move forward with transplantation, for instance.

The V_E/VCO_2 slope is an index of ventilator efficiency and expresses the number of liters of ventilation per liter of CO_2 exhaled. Normal is around <30. High values are a marker of insufficient ventilation due to hyperventilation, increased dead space, or poor gas exchange. High values are expected in heart failure. For instance, in cardiomyopathy a poor prognosis is predicted by values >34.[14]

Cause	Percent
· Hypertrophic cardiomyopathy	26.0
· Anomalous coronary	20.0
· Commotio cordis (direct trauma)	14.0
· Left ventricular hypertrophy	7.5
· Myocarditis	5.0
· Ruptured aortic aneurysm (Marfan syndrome)	3.0
· Arrhythmogenic right ventricular dysplasia	3.0
· Aortic valve stenosis	3.0
All other causes (heat stroke, mitral valve prolapse, dilated cardiomyopathy, long QT, asthma, sarcoidosis, ruptured Berry aneurysm)	13.5

Table 5

Classic Teaching Regarding Causes of Sudden Death in the Young Athlete

Modified from Maron BJ. Sudden death in young athletes. N Engl J Med 2003;349:1064-75.

In patients with adult CHD, the severity of the abnormality of VO_2 max and the VE/VCO_2 slope is dependent on multiple factors, including ventricular function, cyanosis, and pulmonary hypertension. *Figure 4* presents an overview of the impact that the various congenital lesions have on these parameters. Those who do the poorest in this regard include patients with complex anatomy and especially patients with pulmonary hypertension. Those with Eisenmenger syndrome have the worst overall exercise tolerance. As shown in *Figure 4*, the greater the degree of cyanosis, the poorer the response to exercise as well.

Key Point

- A cardiopulmonary exercise test is useful for evaluating the patient with CHD. The two most important measureable parameters are the VO_2 max and the slope of the V_E/CO_2. A low VO_2 max and a very rapid V_E/CO_2 slope imply severe impairment and poor prognosis.

Sudden Cardiac Death

Sudden death in the young athlete is always a newsmaker due to the devastating and unexpected consequences of the event. *Table 5* shows the classic teaching as to the most common causes for sudden death in this situation,[15] the three most common causes are hypertrophic cardiomyopathy, an anomalous coronary (almost always one arising from the opposite coronary cusp and traversing between the PA and aorta), and commotio cordis (direct trauma).

In patients with TOF, the QRS duration has generally been thought to predict those most susceptible to sudden death; a QRS duration >180 msec occurs more likely in those experiencing sudden death in this disease.[16] In TOF, the more dilated the RV, the greater the QRS width, and because many who have undergone tetralogy repair have severe residual low-pressure pulmonary regurgitation, the indication to replace the pulmonary valve is focused on these increased RV dimensions.[17]

Figures 5a, b, and *c* depict the data from recent reviews comparing the causes of sudden death in the young athlete with the general population and adults with CHD. In these reviews, the majority of athletes and the general population who experience sudden death had no clear explanation (this is particularly true in the general population) (*Figure 5a*).[18-20] In adults with CHD, it is very much a mixed bag, with more than half the cases involving Eisenmenger syndrome, congenitally corrected transposition (L-transposition of the great arteries), TOF, or LV outflow tract lesions. Eleven percent of patients had a Fontan procedure and a similar number suffered from Ebstein's anomaly (displacement of the septal and posterior tricuspid valve leaflets into the RV) (*Figure 5b*). QRS duration or QT dispersion did not reveal any clear cutoff value predictive of sudden death in this more recent series (*Figure 5c*).

Because most sudden-death episodes occur during exercise stress, vigorous exercise is discouraged in

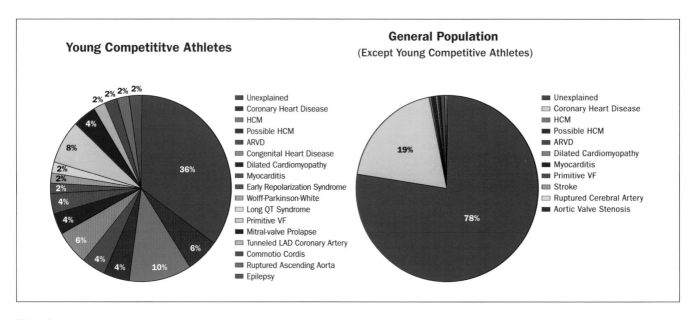

Figure 5a

Comparison of Causes of Sudden Death in Young Competitive Athletes, the General Population, and Adults With CHD

The causes of sudden death in young, competitive athletes are compared with the age-similar causes in the general population. A high percentage of sudden death is unexplained.

ARVD = arrhythmogenic right ventricular dysplasia; HCM = hypertrophic cardiomyopathy; LAD = left anterior descending; VF = ventricular fibrillation.

Reproduced with permission from Marijon E, Tafflet M, Celermajer DS, et al. Sports-related sudden death in the general population. Circulation 2011;124:672-81.

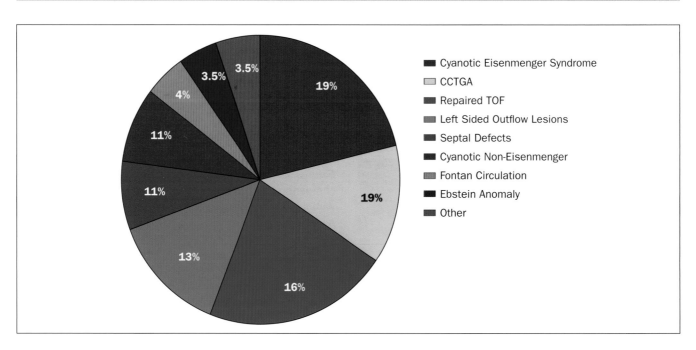

Figure 5b

Comparison of Causes of Sudden Death in Young Competitive Athletes, the General Population, and Adults With CHD

The causes of sudden death in only adults with congenital heart disease.

CCTGA = congenitally corrected transposition of the great arteries; TOF = tetralogy of Fallot.

Reproduced with permission from Koyak Z, Harrix L, de Groot JR, et al. Sudden cardiac death in adult congenital heart disease. Circulation 2012;126:1944-54.

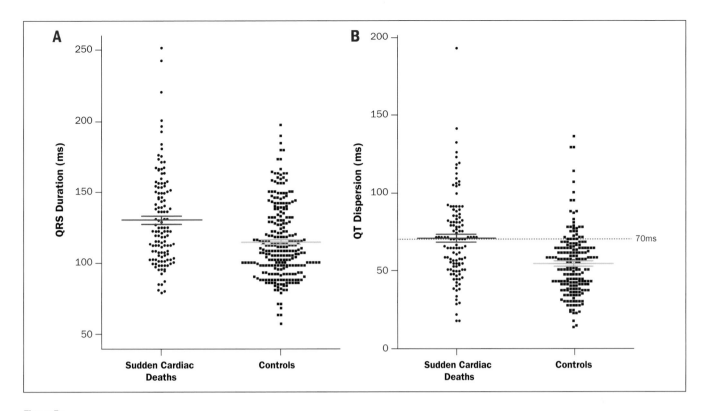

Figure 5c

Comparison of Causes of Sudden Death in Young Competitive Athletes, the General Population, and Adults With CHD

The relationship of the QRS width (**panel A**) and QT dispersion (**panel B**) for the diseases shown in *Figure 5b*. No clear cutoff value associated with sudden death is revealed.

Reproduced with permission from Koyak Z, Harrix L, de Groot JR, et al. Sudden cardiac death in adult congenital heart disease. Circulation 2012;126:1944-54.

patients with obstructive outflow tract lesions and poor ventricular function. The Italian Cardiological Guidelines for Sports Eligibility in Athletes With Heart Disease[21,22] presents a more detailed discussion regarding recommendations for individual lesions.

> **Key Point**
>
> - Although coronary anomalies (especially the left main or left anterior descending between the PA and aorta) remain among the greatest risk factors for sudden death in the young patients, the most common cause is frequently unknown. Those with pulmonary hypertension, a systemic RV, TOF, or LV outflow tract lesions are at great risk as well.

Management of Cardiovascular Risk Factors

As the patient with CHD ages, the impact of vascular disease, systemic hypertension, diabetes, and hyperlipidemia may all become additive to the underlying congenital heart defect. In most cases, these can be managed as with any other patient (although blood pressure management can be complicated, because

lowering systemic resistance can increase a right-to-left shunt, if present). The desire for pregnancy can also impact the treatment options, as do either associated liver or renal impairment.

Heart Failure Management

Heart failure management is generally similar to that of adult patients with cardiomyopathy; although there are fewer clinical trials than those with either systolic and/or diastolic heart failure due to cardiomyopathy, the results often have been less impressive in the adult congenital population.[1] This is particularly true for patients where the RV is primarily involved. For that reason, cardiac resynchronization or multisite pacing still must be considered investigational.[1]

Many challenges also remain regarding heart transplantation suitability. Some of these are psychosocial and economic, some are purely anatomical in regard to replacing the heart or heart/lung due to body habitus or prior interventions, some are complicated by the presence of multiorgan dysfunction, and, finally, some of the problem may relate to a high number of antibodies present due to multiple preceding surgical interventions. All of these factors play a role in determining whether

Intra-atrial Re-entrant Tachycardia
• Around patches, scars, incisions
• Atrial septal defects, tetralogy of Fallot, s/p Mustard or Senning procedure in D-transposition of the great arteries, Fontan procedure
Atrial Fibrillation (*less common than intra-atrial tachycardias*)
• Aortic or mitral valve disease, atrial septal defects, single ventricle
Wolff-Parkinson-White Syndrome
• Ebstein's anomaly
Ventricular Tachycardia
• Repaired tetralogy of Fallot
Sinus Node Dysfunction
• Sinus venosus atrial septal defects, s/p Mustard or Senning in D-transposition of the great arteries, Fontan procedure
AV Nodal Block
• L-transposition (congenitally corrected transposition of the great arteries), atrioventricular septal defect

Table 6

Common Arrhythmias and Frequently Associated Congenital Heart Disease

Reproduced with permission from Bhatt AB, Foster E, Kuehl K, et al. Congenital heart disease in the older adult: a scientific statement from the American Heart Association. Circulation 2015;131:1884-931.

any individual adult congenital patient is suitable for transplantation when the palliative surgical repair is no longer capable of sustaining the patient's clinical status.

Associated Arrhythmias, Pacemaker, and Implantable Cardioverter-Defibrillator Issues

There are certain "classic" arrhythmias associated with congenital heart defects. *Table 6* provides a quick reference to the arrhythmia and its commonly associated cardiac abnormality.[1] In general, intra-atrial re-entrant tachycardias tend to be more common than atrial fibrillation. Often they are associated with re-entry foci near patches, scars, or incisions on the myocardium. This includes patients who have had an ASD repair, TOF repair, Fontan repair, or atrial switch procedure (Mustard or Senning procedures in D-TGA). Atrial fibrillation is more likely to be seen when there is aortic or mitral valve disease or in patients with a single ventricle.

Wolff-Parkinson-White syndrome (pre-excitation) accompanies the Ebstein's valve anomaly in about 15% of cases. Patients with an Ebstein-like anomaly who have L-transposition (congenitally corrected transposition) may have a left-sided appearing Wolff-Parkinson-White pathway.

Ventricular arrhythmias can be associated with any patient with evidence for ventricular dysfunction, but they are particularly common in patients with TOF (frequently from the myocardium adjacent to the RV outflow patch). The sinus node sits epicardially at the junction of the SVC and RA, and, as expected, sinus node dysfunction is common in patients with a superior sinus venosus ASD (where a low atrial rhythm is occasionally present) or whenever there is surgical intervention in the area of the sinus node (such as after sinus venosus repair, following a Glenn procedure, or after the Mustard or Senning atrial switch operations).

Finally, because of inherently abnormal AV nodal architecture, AV block is common in patients who have transposition of the great arteries or those with an AV septal defect. In L-transposition, the mantra of expecting a 2% per year incidence of heart block has become a clinical expectation.

At times, the most difficult decision regarding pacemaker implantation relates to whether there is appropriate venous access. For instance, in patients with dual SVC systems (persistent left SVC) there may or may not be a connector (innominate) vein between the two SVC. Also, placing a pacemaker in the venous system of a patient with a right-to-left shunt increases the possibility of an embolic stroke. Pacer placement within the baffles of a patient with a Mustard or Senning atrial switch not infrequently results in baffle stenosis. This latter can lead to baffle obstruction and/or a baffle leak and then cyanosis. Most guidelines recommend that dual chamber pacing be maintained if at all possible. In addition, before considering biventricular pacing or defibrillator implantation, any outstanding hemodynamic issue should first be corrected. Epicardial leads and, more recently, subcutaneous defibrillators may reduce the risk for intracardiac thrombosis.

Pulmonary Hypertension and Eisenmenger Syndrome

Pulmonary hypertension is defined as a resting mean PA pressure of >25 mm Hg, that when related to CHD falls into the World Health Organization Group 1 category.[23-25] Pulmonary hypertension in patients with CHD is much more likely to occur when there is a significant left-to-right shunt and the lesion is distal to the tricuspid valve (ventricular septal defect, patent ductus arteriosus). In some patients, subpulmonic or pulmonic valve stenosis may be protective of the pulmonary circuit and patients live for many years

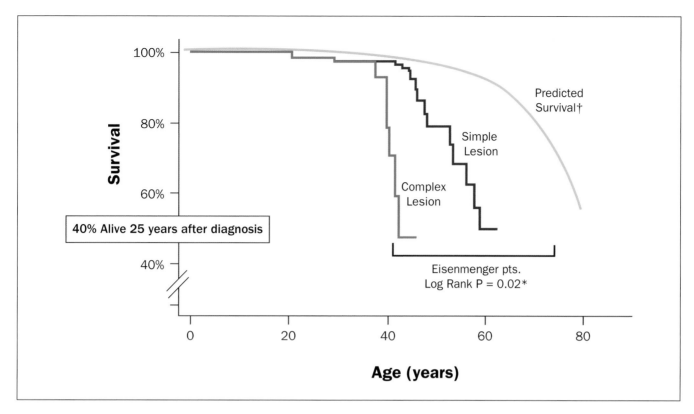

Figure 6

Long-Term Outcomes in Patients With Eisenmenger Syndrome

Complex lesions with Eisenmenger syndrome do well until about of 40 years of age. Less complex lesions with Eisemenger syndrome start to decline later and the falloff is more gradual.

†Predicted survival is based on the life tables for UK and Wales (2001–2003 interim life tables) published by the Government Actuary's Department.

*Comparison between Eisenmenger patients with simple and complex lesions. Patients with complex lesions had a significantly worse outcome compared with those with simple lesions.

Reproduced with permission from Diller GP, Dimopoulos K, Broberg CS, et al. Presentation, survival prospects, and predictors of death in Eisenmenger syndrome: a combined retrospective and case-control study. Eur Heart J 2006;27:1737-42.

without surgical correction. Only about 10-15% of patients with shunts proximal to the tricuspid valve (ASD, anomalous pulmonary veins) develop pulmonary hypertension, and many of these are associated with repair of the defect late in life. Occasionally, pulmonary hypertension can develop even after a cardiac shunt has been effectively closed.

The degree of pulmonary hypertension often determines whether a shunt is considered repairable if the two lesions are present. As a generality, whenever the PA pressure/systemic pressure is >2/3, the shunt is considered inoperable. Vasodilator therapy may be used to bring the pressures down to meet operability goals (as long as there is persistence of a left-to-right shunt).

Eisenmenger syndrome is defined as pulmonary hypertension with cyanosis (right-to-left shunting). Survival in patients with Eisenmenger physiology is much better than that of idiopathic pulmonary hypertension (*Figure 6*). In fact, 40% of patients with Eisenmenger

pulmonary hypertension are alive fully 25 years after the diagnosis has been made.[25]

Patients with Eisenmenger physiology are rarely considered operable and their management revolves around the prevention of complications. *Table 7* outlines the major complications one should monitor in these patients. Cyanosis triggers the bone marrow to increase the red blood cell (RBC) mass and hematocrits can reach over 70% at times. This can lead to sledging in the small vessels and the hyperviscosity syndrome. Patients often complain of headaches, muscle cramps, nausea, and abdominal pain. Patients with Eisenmenger physiology and a patent ductus arteriosus may experience reversal of the shunt at the patent ductus arteriosus with desaturated blood going to the lower extremities. This can result in cyanosis and clubbing of the feet while the hands remain pink (differential cyanosis).

Iron deficiency alters the size and shape of the RBCs and is known to increase the risk for symptomatic hyperviscosity.

- Hyperviscosity
- Bleeding and hemoptysis
- Air or thrombus emboli
- Congestive heart failure
- Hyperuricemia (gout, renal dysfunction, renal calculi)
- Calcium bilirubinate gallstones
- Infections
- Hypertrophic cardiomyopathy

Table 7

Potential Complications and Important Monitoring Studies in Patients With Eisenmenger Physiology

Patients should therefore have their ferritin checked yearly and phlebotomies done only for symptoms. The mean RBC volume may not reflect the presence of iron deficiency due to an increase in immature macrocytic RBCs in the blood stream, so it should be monitored. If iron deficiency is present, a short course of supplemental iron (usually over 1 month) should be administered until the ferritin is normal. Iron loss is frequently due to bleeding in the gastrointestinal tract.

Hemoptysis from ruptured bronchial vessels is a concern as well; the larger of these vessels can be coil occluded when necessary. Patients with Eisenmenger physiology also tend to be hypercoagulable and in-situ thrombus is common in the markedly dilated pulmonary arteries that are present. Because, by definition, there is right-to-left shunting, there is also the risk for paradoxical emboli and many patients will require anticoagulation unless there is evidence for gastrointestinal bleeding or hemoptysis. These patients are also susceptible to air emboli when admitted to the hospital and filters should always be placed on intravenous (IV) lines to reduce that risk.

Other complications include congestive heart failure, primarily right heart failure as the RV is designed more for volume rather than pressure overload. Arrhythmias, particularly atrial arrhythmias, are frequent and should be appropriately treated. The increased bone marrow activity can result in an increase in uric acid levels and subsequent gout, renal dysfunction, and uric acid renal calculi. Calcium bilirubinate gallstones (black stones) may also occur and trigger acute cholecystitis. Elevated right heart pressures may result in cirrhosis. Right-to-left shunting also sets the stage for cerebral abscess formation. As with others with lung disease, a hypertrophic osteoarthropathy (increased density at the ends of long bones) may occur.

Table 8 outlines therapeutic options for patients with Eisenmenger syndrome. Prophylactic options include night-time oxygen therapy, although often the right-to-left shunting precludes any improvement in the arterial

Prophylactic Measures
- Oxygen? Some suggest at night only
- Filters on all intravenous lines
- Avoidance of pregnancy, extreme exercise, high altitude, dehydration, anticoagulation (unless high risk without it), tobacco use, intravascular pacemakers

Phlebotomy
- Only for symptoms (occasionally preoperative when hematocrit >65%)

Hydration

Endocarditis prophylaxis

Pulmonary vasodilators

Lung or heart/lung transplantation

Table 8

Therapeutic Options in the Treatment of Eisenmenger Syndrome

Class IIa (LOE B): *Before Dental Procedures*
° Prosthetic cardiac valve or prosthetic material used for cardiac valve repair. ° Previous infective endocarditis. ° Unrepaired and palliated cyanotic congenital heart disease (CHD), including surgically constructed palliative shunts and conduits. ° Completely repaired CHD with prosthetic materials, whether placed by surgery or catheter intervention, during the first 6 months after the procedure. ° Repaired CHD with residual defects at the site or adjacent to the site of a prosthetic patch or prosthetic device that might inhibit endothelialization.
Class IIa (LOE C): *At time of Membrane Rupture Before Vaginal Delivery*
° Prosthetic cardiac valve or prosthetic material used for cardiac valve repair. ° Unrepaired and palliated cyanotic CHD, including surgically constructed palliative shunts and conduits.
Class III (LOE C)
° No endocarditis prophylaxis recommended for nondental procedures *in the absence of active infection.*

Table 9

Antibiotic Prophylaxis During Procedures in Adults With Congenital Heart Disease

LOE = Level of Evidence.

Reproduced with permission from Warnes CA, Williams RG, Bashore TM, et al. ACC/AHA 2008 guidelines for the management of adults with congenital heart disease: a report of the American College of Cardiology/American Heart Association Task Force on Practice Guidelines (Writing Committee to Develop Guidelines on the Management of Adults With Congenital Heart Disease). Developed in collaboration with the American Society of Echocardiography, Heart Rhythm Society, International Society for Adult Congenital Heart Disease, Society for Cardiovascular Angiography and Interventions, and Society of Thoracic Surgeons. J Am Coll Cardiol 2008;52:e143-263.

oxygen saturations. As mentioned, all IVs should have filters. Patients should avoid pregnancy, extreme exercise, high altitude exposure, dehydration, and tobacco abuse. Anticoagulation carries a risk, and its use should be a case-by-case risk/benefit decision.

The hyperviscosity syndrome is treated with phlebotomy. It is important to replace any blood removed with a similar volume of normal saline. Phlebotomy should be reserved for symptom relief only, although some advocate for phlebotomy prior to noncardiac surgeries when the hematocrit exceeds 65%. Endocarditis prophylaxis is recommended, as infective endocarditis can be life-threatening and surgical options may be few. Whether it is effective or not remains an open question, but all guidelines continue to recommend its usage.

Pulmonary vasodilators can improve exercise tolerance and often oxygen saturations, although there are no data on improvement of long-term survival.[1,26] Calcium blockers may not be tolerated due to RV dysfunction and phosphodiesterase-5 inhibitors (i.e., sildenafil) are rarely effective. Endothelin receptor blockers and prostanoids can improve clinical status as long as systemic vasodilation is avoided (as right-to-left shunting may increase). In many instances, the only viable long-term option is to consider lung transplantation and cardiac repair, or heart-lung transplant. As noted earlier, these patients frequently present a challenge when considering transplantation options.

Infective Endocarditis

Adult patients with CHD are susceptible to infective endocarditis. Because the initial lesion in this process is endothelial injury, any lesion that might disrupt the endothelium (including jet lesions from high-pressure to low-pressure chambers or vessels) could become a focus for infective endocarditis. Although rare, the hemodynamic consequences of the infection and the underlying congenital disease can make treatment options difficult. The ACC/AHA 2008 Guidelines for the Management of Adults With Congenital Heart Disease[2] expanded on the AHA/ACC Guideline for the Management of Patients With Valvular Heart Disease[27-29] by including prophylactic coverage during vaginal delivery. *Table 9* outlines the current recommendations for whom to cover for prophylaxis in this patient population.

- Heart failure treatment that has been proven effective in adults with cardiomyopathy may not always prove effective in adults with CHD. RV dysfunction (regardless of whether it is the pulmonary or the systemic ventricle) appears to respond less well to conventional treatment for LV dysfunction.

- Transplantation may be the only long-term option for some patients with congenital disease. This is complicated by psychosocial issues, economic issues, anatomic concerns, body habitus, the presence of multiorgan dysfunction, and the presence of a high number of antibodies from multiple prior surgeries.

- Certain arrhythmias are particularly associated with certain CHD. These include Wolff-Parkinson-White syndrome and Ebstein's anomaly, complete heart block and L-transposition of the great arteries, ventricular arrhythmias and TOF outflow patch areas, sinus node dysfunction and sinus venosus repair, or the Glenn/Fontan procedure.

- Intra-atrial re-entry tachycardias are generally more frequent in patients with CHD than is atrial fibrillation.

- Eisenmenger syndrome is defined by the presence of pulmonary hypertension (mean PA >25 mm Hg at rest) and right-to-left shunting. It is much more common in intracardiac shunts distal to the tricuspid valve.

- Forty percent of patients with Eisenmenger syndrome live at least 25 years after the diagnosis.

- Patients with Eisenmenger syndrome should have yearly measures of the hematocrit, uric acid, and ferritin.

- Patients with Eisenmenger physiology and a patent ductus arteriosus will have differential cyanosis with pink nails on the upper extremity and cyanosis and clubbing of both feet. This is due to reversal of the shunt at the patent ductus arteriosus.

- In patients with Eisenmenger syndrome, phlebotomy should not be performed unless there are symptoms of hyperviscosity. Some suggest that phlebotomy may be considered if the hematocrit is >65% prior to noncardiac surgery. Iron may be given over a short course if the ferritin is low to reduce hyperviscosity.

- Because of the right-to-left shunting in Eisenmenger patients, pacemaker leads can present a risk if thrombus formation occurs. IV fluids should always have filters placed to prevent air emboli.

- Pulmonary vasodilators have been shown to improve arterial saturation and symptoms, but not survival, in Eisenmenger patients.

- Prophylaxis for the prevention of endocarditis applies to many patients with CHD, and the recommendations suggest coverage during vaginal delivery if the patient is at high risk.

References

1. Bhatt AB, Foster E, Kuehl K, et al. Congenital heart disease in the older adult: a scientific statement from the American Heart Association. Circulation 2015;131:1884-931.

2. Warnes CA, Williams RG, Bashore TM, et al. ACC/AHA 2008 guidelines for the management of adults with congenital heart disease: a report of the American College of Cardiology/American Heart Association Task Force on Practice Guidelines (Writing Committee to Develop Guidelines on the Management of Adults With Congenital Heart Disease). Developed in collaboration with the American Society of Echocardiography, Heart Rhythm Society, International Society for Adult Congenital Heart Disease, Society for Cardiovascular Angiography and Interventions, and Society of Thoracic Surgeons. J Am Coll Cardiol 2008;52:e143-263.

3. Kaltman JR, Andropoulos DB, Checchia PA, et al. Report of the Pediatric Heart Network and National Heart, Lung, and Blood Institute Working Group on the Perioperative Management of Congenital Heart Disease. Circulation 2010;121:2766-72.

4. Marelli AJ, Mackie AS, Ionescu-Ittu R, Rahme E, Pilote L. Congenital heart disease in the general population: changing prevalence and age distribution. Circulation 2007;115:163-72.

5. Silversides CK, Marelli A, Beauchesne L, et al. Canadian Cardiovascular Society 2009 Consensus Conference on the management of adults with congenital heart disease: executive summary. Can J Cardiol 2010;26:143-50.

6. Baumgartner H, Bonhoeffer P, De Groot NM, et al. ESC Guidelines for the management of grown-up congenital heart disease (new version 2010). Eur Heart J 2010;31:2915-57.

7. Lin AE, Basson CT, Goldmuntz E, et al. Adults with genetic syndromes and cardiovascular abnormalities: clinical history and management. Genet Med 2008;10:469-94.

8. Biner S, Rafique AM, Ray I, Cuk O, Siegel RJ, Tolstrup K. Aortopathy is prevalent in relatives of bicuspid aortic valve patients. J Am Coll Cardiol 2009;53:2288-95.

9. Potter BJ, Leong-Sit P, Fernandes SM, et al. Effect of aspirin and warfarin therapy on thromboembolic events in patients with univentricular hearts and Fontan palliation. Int J Cardiol 2013;168:3940-3.

10. Ohuchi H, Yasuda K, Miyazaki A, et al. Prevalence and predictors of haemostatic complications in 412 Fontan patients: their relation to anticoagulation and haemodynamics. Eur J Cardiothorac Surg 2015;47:511-9.

11. Elder RW, Parekh S, Book WM. More on hepatocellular carcinoma after the Fontan procedure. N Engl J Med 2013;369:490.

12. Schumacher KR, Gossett J, Guleserian K, et al. Fontan-associated protein-losing enteropathy and heart transplant: a Pediatric Heart Transplant Study analysis. J Heart Lung Transplant 2015;34:1169-76.

13. Balady GJ, Arena R, Sietsema K, et al. Clinician's guide to cardio-pulmonary exercise testing in adults: a scientific statement from the American Heart Association. Circulation 2010;122:191-225.

14. Chua TP, Ponikowski P, Harrington D, et al. Clinical correlates and prognostic significance of the ventilatory response to exercise in chronic heart failure. J Am Coll Cardiol 1997;29:1585-90.

15. Maron BJ. Sudden death in young athletes. N Engl J Med 2003;349:1064-75.

16. Gatzoulis MA, Till JA, Somerville J, Redington AN. Mechano-electrical interaction in tetralogy of Fallot. QRS prolongation relates to right ventricular size and predicts malignant ventricular arrhythmias and sudden death. Circulation 1995;92:231-7.

17. Lewis MJ, O'Connor DS, Rozenshtien A, et al. Usefulness of magnetic resonance imaging to guide referral for pulmonary valve replacement in repaired tetralogy of Fallot. Am J Cardiol 2014;114:1406-11.

18. Marijon E, Tafflet M, Celermajer DS, et al. Sports-related sudden death in the general population. Circulation 2011;124:672-81.

19. Estes NA 3rd. Predicting and preventing sudden cardiac death. Circulation 2011;124:651-6.

20. Link MS, Estes NA 3rd. Sudden cardiac death in the athlete: bridging the gaps between evidence, policy, and practice. Circulation 2012;125:2511-6.

21. Biffi A, Delise P, Zeppilli P, et al. Italian cardiological guidelines for sports eligibility in athletes with heart disease: part 2. J Cardiovasc Med (Hagerstown) 2013;14:500-15.

22. Biffi A, Delise P, Zeppilli P, et al. Italian cardiological guidelines for sports eligibility in athletes with heart disease: part 1. J Cardiovasc Med (Hagerstown) 2013;14:477-99.

23. Rose ML, Strange G, King I, et al. Congenital heart disease-associated pulmonary arterial hypertension: preliminary results from a novel registry. Intern Med J 2012;42:874-9.

24. Galie N, Corris PA, Frost A, et al. Updated treatment algorithm of pulmonary arterial hypertension. J Am Coll Cardiol 2013;62:D60-72.

25. Diller GP, Dimopoulos K, Broberg CS, et al. Presentation, survival prospects, and predictors of death in Eisenmenger syndrome: a combined retrospective and case-control study. Eur Heart J 2006;27:1737-42.

26. Rose-Jones LJ, McLaughlin VV. Pulmonary hypertension: types and treatments. Curr Cardiol Rev 2015;11:73-9.

27. Nishimura RA, Otto CM, Bonow RO, et al. 2014 AHA/ACC guideline for the management of patients with valvular heart disease: a report of the American College of Cardiology/American Heart Association Task Force on Practice Guidelines. J Am Coll Cardiol 2014;63:e57-185.

28. Bach DS, American College of Cardiology/American Heart Association. Perspectives on the American College of Cardiology/American Heart Association guidelines for the prevention of infective endocarditis. J Am Coll Cardiol 2009;53:1852-4.

29. Pant S, Patel NJ, Deshmukh A, et al. Trends in infective endocarditis incidence, microbiology, and valve replacement in the United States from 2000 to 2011. J Am Coll Cardiol 2015;65:2070-6.

Congenital Heart Disease

Pretricuspid Valve Shunts

Shunt Lesions

Intracardiac shunts are the most common form of congenital heart lesions and are frequently diagnosed in otherwise healthy adults. Under normal conditions, the blood flowing to the pulmonary arterial vascular bed should have the same oxygen saturation as the mixture of blood returning to the right atrium (RA). When this is not the case, a left-to-right shunt is said to be present, and an increase in saturation or "step-up" is noted downstream from the abnormal communication. Flow through such lesions is generally dependent on two main features: 1) the size of the lesion, and 2) the difference in compliance between the pulmonary and the systemic circuits.

Although echocardiographic techniques can roughly estimate the degree of shunting, the most accurate calculation of shunt fraction requires cardiac catheterization. A shunt is quantified during catheterization by examining the blood oxygen saturations in the respective chambers.

The mixed venous (MV) saturation is the saturation of blood returning to the RA and has contributions from the inferior vena cava (IVC), superior vena cava (SVC), and coronary sinus (CS). IVC saturation is normally higher than the SVC because of high renal blood flow and less oxygen extraction by the kidney. The CS saturation is very low, but its volume of contribution is negligible and usually ignored. To normalize the MV saturation, three times the SVC saturation is added to the IVC saturation, and the sum is then divided by four.

Because so much mixing of blood with differing saturations occurs in the RA, an 11% increase in oxygen saturation is required to diagnose a shunt lesion between the vena cavae and the RA, a 7% increase is necessary to detect a shunt between the RA and right ventricle (RV), and a 5% increase is needed to detect a shunt between the RV and pulmonary artery (PA). A quick and simple measure of the overall size of a left-to-right shunt ratio can be obtained by using this formula: aortic saturation–MV saturation/ pulmonary vein (PV) saturation–PA saturation).The PV saturation generally is assumed to be 97% if not directly measured.

If a shunt goes unrepaired, the chambers downstream from the lesion can become dilated from the excessive blood flow. This increases the risk of atrial and possibly ventricular arrhythmias as well, depending on the lesion location and size. A less well understood complication of shunts is the development of pulmonary vascular disease (pulmonary arterial hypertension [PAH]).[1] About 5-10% of patients will develop PAH, with post-tricuspid valve lesions (such as a ventricular septal defect [VSD] or patent ductus arteriosus) much more commonly leading to this complication.

When PAH occurs, the shunt fraction may be reduced. When pulmonary vascular resistance (PVR) exceeds systemic resistance, shunt flow can reverse, defining the Eisenmenger syndrome.The latter occurs in 35-50% of patients with shunt lesions and PAH. In Eisenmenger syndrome, shunting becomes right-to-left and systemic oxygenation decreases. In addition, the saturation will not normalize when oxygen is administered

Richard A. Krasuski, MD, FACC
Consultant Fees/Honoraria: Actelion Pharmaceuticals, Ventripoint, Bayer Healthcare Pharmaceuticals; Speaker's Bureau: Actelion Pharmaceuticals.

Learner Objectives

Upon completion of this module, the reader will be able to:
1. Identify the complications that result from unrepaired intracardiac shunts and describe methods of diagnosis, quantification, and correction.
2. Differentiate between a patent foramen ovale (PFO) and an atrial septal defect (ASD) and recognize what constitutes a significant ASD.
3. Recognize the difficulty in detecting partial anomalous pulmonary venous return (PAPVR).

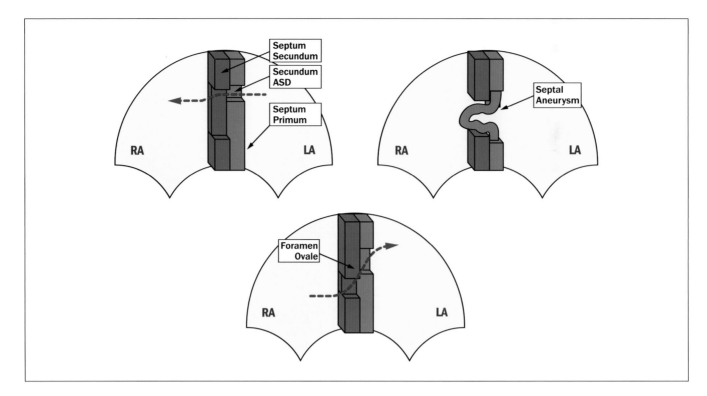

Figure 1
Variations in Septal Anatomy

ASD = atrial septal defect; LA = left atrium; RA = right atrium.

Modified from Krasuski RA, Bashore TM. The emerging role of percutaneous intervention in adults with congenital heart disease. Rev Cardiovasc Med 2005;6:11-22.

as the shunt flow does not pass through the lungs. Multiple complications eventually ensue, and until recently, this condition was considered irreversible. Another condition associated with ASD is stroke, which presumably results from paradoxical embolization (blood clots forming in the extremities and reaching the cerebral circulation by passing through the ASD).

Key Points

- About 5-10% of patients with shunt lesions develop PAH, with post-tricuspid valve lesions more commonly leading to this complication.

- About 35-50% of patients with unrepaired shunt lesions and PAH will develop Eisenmenger syndrome (shunt reversal as a result of pulmonary vascular disease resulting in hypoxic complications).

Atrial Septal Development

To facilitate understanding of the various abnormalities in the atrial septum (*Figure 1*), it is important to first review its embryologic development (*Video 1*). The heart starts

 Video - not available for print.

Video 1
Process of Atrial Septation

The septum primum and secundum sequentially form from the roof of the common atrium. Just before birth the foramen ovale remains patent to facilitate blood bypassing the pulmonary circuit.

out with a single atrium. During early development, the septum primum starts growing downward from the roof of this chamber and divides the atrium into a left and a right side. Fenestrations eventually form in the middle of the septum primum, creating the ostium secundum (*Figure 2*). A second septum (the septum secundum) then develops on the right atrial side of the septum primum. At the completion of normal formation of the septum secundum, an opening (or flap) referred to as the "foramen ovale" still remains. This structure functions as a one-way (right-to-left) valve to provide a passageway for blood to bypass the lungs in utero.[2]

At birth, the lung pressures drop and the blood pressure in the left atrium (LA) exceeds that of the RA, leading to

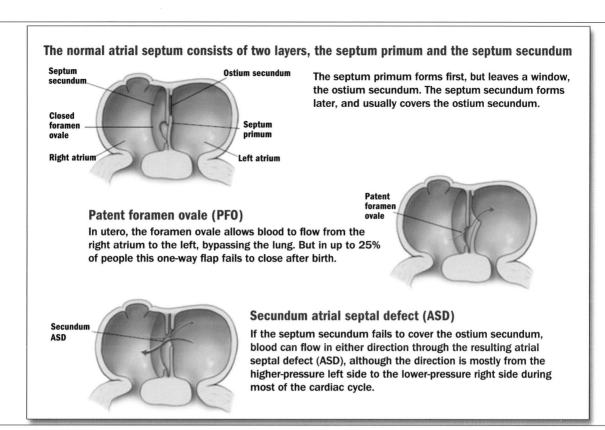

The normal atrial septum consists of two layers, the septum primum and the septum secundum

Septum secundum

Ostium secundum

Closed foramen ovale

Septum primum

Right atrium

Left atrium

The septum primum forms first, but leaves a window, the ostium secundum. The septum secundum forms later, and usually covers the ostium secundum.

Patent foramen ovale (PFO)

In utero, the foramen ovale allows blood to flow from the right atrium to the left, bypassing the lung. But in up to 25% of people this one-way flap fails to close after birth.

Patent foramen ovale

Secundum atrial septal defect (ASD)

If the septum secundum fails to cover the ostium secundum, blood can flow in either direction through the resulting atrial septal defect (ASD), although the direction is mostly from the higher-pressure left side to the lower-pressure right side during most of the cardiac cycle.

Secundum ASD

Figure 2
Holes in the Heart: Two Main Types

apposition of the septum and complete sealing of the defect within hours of birth in up to 75% of infants. If the final step does not occur, a PFO remains present. In general, such a lesion should mainly result in the potential for right-to-left and not left-to-right shunting, as occurs when the right atrial pressure exceeds that of the LA, such as during a Valsalva maneuver or general straining (*Video 2*).

The septum secundum will completely cover the opening fenestration in the septum primum >99% of the time. If it fails to properly develop, however, the result is a secundum ASD, which is a hole in the septum that permits blood to flow in either direction (left-to-right or right-to-left; *Video 3*), depending on the atrial pressures. This is the most common type of ASD (*Figure 3*). More complicated defects of the septum include the sinus venosus ASD, which forms at the junction of the SVC or IVC and the RA. This type of defect is commonly associated with abnormalities in blood return from the lungs (anomalous pulmonary venous return). Even rarer are the primum ASDs or atrioventricular (AV) canal defects, which also involve the AV (mitral and tricuspid) valves.

Patent Foramen Ovale

PFO is a very common lesion, occurring in approximately 25% of the general population. Unlike an ASD, a PFO does not result in left-to-right shunt or its complications

(*Table 1*). In most patients, a PFO will never be associated with any problems. This makes attribution of pathologies to this lesion difficult and controversial. The prevalence of a PFO was previously thought to decrease in older patients, implying that patients with a PFO tended to die young or

Video - not available for print.

Video 2
Bubble Study Using Biatrial View on Transesopheageal Echo

Bubbles injected into the venous circulation cross from the right atrium (bottom of the screen) to the left atrium (top of the screen) through the foramen tunnel.

Video - not available for print.

Video 3
Subcostal Echo View of ASD Using Color Doppler

A subcostal image using color Doppler demonstrates color flow that mostly consists of left-to-right shunting (from the left atrium bottom of the screen to the right atrium at the top).

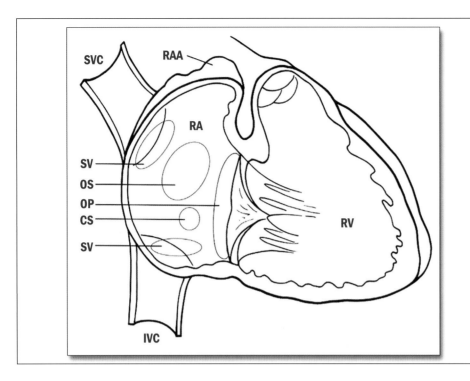

Figure 3
Types of Atrial Septal Defects

Ostium secundum (OS) is centrally located and most common. Ostium primum (OP) involves atrial and ventricular septa and often valves as well. Sinus venosus (SV) can be superior or inferior and has associated anomalous pulmonary veins. Coronary sinus (CS) is least common.

IVC = inferior vena cava; RA = right atrium; RAA = right atrial appendage; RV = right ventricle; SVC = superior vena cava.

Atrial Septal Defect	Patent Foramen Ovale
Incidence approximately 1/600	Incidence approximately 1/4
Usually left-to-right shunt	Usually only right-to-left shunt
Also has right-to-left shunt	"Stretched PFO" can result in left-to-right shunt
Association with stroke	Association with stroke
Can be concurrent with ASA	Can be concurrent with ASA
Results in "flow" complications · Right heart enlargement · Pulmonary hypertension · Atrial fibrillation	No "flow" complications

Table 1
Atrial Septal Defect Versus Patent Foramen Ovale

ASA = atrial septal aneurysm; PFO = patent foramen ovale.

that spontaneous closure occurred later in life, but these data now have been refuted.[3]

The pathological importance of a PFO is controversial, and what to do when a PFO is found during routine clinical imaging remains unclear. In healthy populations, a PFO does not independently predict future stroke risk.[4] Most studies suggesting associations of pathology with PFO have been cohort studies comparing the prevalence of PFO in index cases and controls. These have drawn associations between a PFO and several disease processes, including stroke and transient ischemic attack (TIA), migraine headaches, decompression sickness, platypnea-orthodeoxia (a condition defined by shortness of breath in which systemic levels of oxygen drop on sitting or standing after a recumbent position) and provoked exercise desaturation (drop in arterial oxygen saturation with stair climbing).[5]

Prior cohort studies suggested a potential role for percutaneous closure of PFO to reduce recurrent stroke

Study	Device Used	Number of Patients	Mean Age (years)	Randomization (device vs. medications)	Medical Therapies (some treated with both agents)	Mean Follow-up (years)	Strokes (device vs. meds)	P-Value
CLOSURE I	Cardioseal	909	46.0	1:1	66% antiplatelet 34% anticoagulant		12 vs. 13 (at 2 years)	0.79
RESPECT	Amplatzer septal occluder	980	45.9	1:1	75% antiplatelet 25% anticoagulant	2.6 ± 2.0	9 vs. 16	0.08
PC	Amplatzer septal occluder	414	44.5	1:1	74% antiplatelet 31% anticoagulant	4.1 years	1 vs. 7	0.07
REDUCE	Helex	664		2:1				
CLOSE	Multiple	900		1:1				

Table 2
Randomized Studies of Patent Foramen Ovale Following Stroke or Transient Ischemic Attack

and possibly reduce the frequency of migraine headaches. Closure of PFO in patients with recurrent cryptogenic stroke on adequate medical therapy was previously given a Class IIb, Level of Evidence C guideline recommendation,[5] but the management of PFO after a first event is even more controversial. To date, three published trials have randomized patients to either medical therapy or device closure following an initial neurological event. These include CLOSURE I (Safety and Efficacy of the STARFlex Septal Closure System Versus Best Medical Therapy in Patients With a Stroke or TIA due to Presumed Paradoxical Embolism Through a PFO) trial,[6] RESPECT (Randomized Evaluation of Recurrent Stroke Comparing PFO Closure to Established Current Standard of Care Treatment) trial,[7] and PC (Percutaneous Closure) trial.[8] In each study, the rate of subsequent stroke was much lower than expected (between 2-4% over follow-up periods of 2-4 years), and the primary endpoint was not met (*Table 2*). Major procedural complications occurred in 0-4.2% of patients who underwent closure; and in Closure I, the subsequent risk of atrial fibrillation was considerably higher in the device arm. Two additional large studies—REDUCE (Gore Helex Septal Occluder/Gore Septal Occluder for Patent Foramen Ovale Closure in Stroke Patients) study and CLOSE (Patent Foramen Ovale Closure or Anticoagulants Versus Antiplatelet Therapy to Prevent Stroke Recurrence) trial— have recently completed patient recruitment. Of note, the MIST (Migraine Intervention With STARFlex Technology) trial, a randomized, sham procedure-controlled study in migraine patients, also failed to demonstrate significant improvement with device closure.[9] Multiple meta-analyses of the stroke data have been published recently, each with conflicting findings and further increasing the uncertainty of management in this scenario.

Key Points

- PFO occurs in approximately 25% of the population, does not result in left-to-right shunt-related complications, and is only rarely associated with any pathologic sequelae (stroke, migraine, platypnea-orthodeoxia or provoked exercise desaturation).

- Although PFO is more common in patients with cryptogenic stroke than in matched controls, the role of device closure remains uncertain.

Atrial Septal Aneurysm

When there is overabundant and weakened tissue in the septum primum, making the septum very floppy, an atrial septal aneurysm (ASA) is said to be present (*Video 4*). In general, the maximal excursion has to be ≥15 mm (measured from the LA to the RA by echocardiography) for the abnormality to be called an ASA. If the maximal excursion is <15 mm, it generally is referred to as a "redundant atrial septum."

Either a secundum ASD or a PFO can coexist with an ASA. Not surprisingly, a PFO is more likely to be present. In some published series, as many as 60% of patients with PFO have a concomitant ASA. The coexistence of an ASA may increase the probability of recurrent neurological events in patients with atrial-level shunting who present with stroke or TIA.[10]

Video 4

Aneurysmal Atrial Septum on Apical 4-Chamber Echo View

The interatrial septum (bottom of screen) is mobile with full excursion measured to be ~1.5 cm, which meets criteria for an atrial spetal aneurysm.

Video 5

Three-Dimensional View of Oval-Shaped ASD From Right Atrium

The three-dimensional view looking from the right atrium over to the left atrium. The hole seen on the left of the screen is the superior vena cava. The large oval-shaped defect in the middle is the secundum atrial septal defect. To the right of the screen are seen the coronary sinus and inferior vena cava.

Video 6

Fenestrated ASD Visualized With Color Doppler on Intracardiac Echo

The intracardiac echo view of a fenestrated atrial septal defect using color Doppler. The right atrium is at the top of the screen and the left atrium on the bottom. The red flow visualized is passing from the left atrium to right atrium through the multiple defects.

Key Point

- Up to 60% of patients with PFO have a concomitant ASA, which may increase recurrent neurological event risk in patients with stroke or TIA.

Atrial Septal Defects

ASD is the most common congenital heart defect encountered in adults (excluding mitral valve prolapse [MVP] and bicuspid aortic valve), accounting for up to 15% of all adult congenital heart disease. The most common type of ASD (75% of the cases) is the secundum ASD, in which the defect lies in the middle of the atrial septum (*Video 5*). A single defect usually is present, but in up to 10% of patients, more than one defect is present. Occasionally, multiple holes are present (*Video 6*), the so-called "Swiss cheese septum." Almost one-third of patients with ASD will have associated additional malformations such as pulmonary stenosis, VSD, MVP, subaortic stenosis, aortic coarctation, and anomalous pulmonary venous drainage.

The secundum ASD is often mistaken for other abnormalities or is overlooked because the symptoms associated with it, including fatigue, palpitations, and breathlessness, can be subtle and nonspecific. An ASD should be suspected whenever right heart enlargement is present without another good explanation. Physical examination findings, which include a fixed split-second heart sound (as a result of loss of differential effects on right- and left-sided filling pressures from a drop in intrathoracic pressure that normally occurs during inspiration) and a pulmonary outflow murmur (the result of increased pulmonary blood volume from shunting), also may be overlooked.

On electrocardiography, an incomplete right bundle branch block, right axis deviation, abnormal P-wave axis, and right atrial enlargement are commonly seen. *Table 3* compares the clinical and electrocardiographic findings in the most common types of ASD. On chest X-ray, prominent pulmonary arteries, right atrial and ventricular enlargement, and pulmonary plethora can be seen.

The larger the left-to-right shunt in patients with ASD, the greater the risk for long-term complications, such as atrial fibrillation (typically in the fifth decade) and pulmonary hypertension. The latter condition affects up to 5-10% of adults with ASD and if uncorrected can result in Eisenmenger syndrome (*Video 7*). In this syndrome, the right-sided pressure increases to the point that shunting is reversed (becoming right to left) and systemic oxygenation decreases. Patients with this complication will not significantly improve their oxygen saturation when oxygen is administered to them (the telltale sign of a right-to-left shunt). Multiple complications eventually ensue, and until recently, this condition was considered irreversible. There is now growing data that medical management of pulmonary hypertension can lead to symptomatic improvement and possibly improve long-term survival in this high-risk patient population.[1]

Video 7

Large ASD With Right-Sided Enlargement on Cardiac MRI 4-Chamber View

This 4-chamber MRI view shows the very large secundum atrial septal defect (on the left side of the image) with severe right atrial and right ventricular enlargement (on the upper half of the image) due to the development of severe pulmonary hypertension and Eisenmenger syndrome.

	Secundum ASD	Primum ASD	Sinus Venosus ASD
Unique Anatomical Features	PAPVR (only approximately 10%)	1. Mitral valve involvement 2. ± VSD	PAPVR
Physical Exam Findings	1. Fixed split S_2 2. Pulmonary outflow murmur	1. Same as secundum ASD 2. Murmurs of MR ± VSD	Same as secundum ASD
ECG	1. RSR' pattern 2. Incomplete RBBB 3. ± Right axis	1. RBBB 2. Left axis 3. ± First-degree AV block	1. Same as secundum 2. ± Leftward shifted P-wave axis (inverted P in lead III)

Table 3

Unique Features of the Atrial Septal Defects

ASD = atrial septal defect; AV = atrioventricular; ECG = electrocardiogram; MR = mitral regurgitation; PAPVR = partial anomalous pulmonary venous return; RBBB = right bundle branch block; S_2 = second heart sound; VSD = ventricular septal defect.

The American College of Cardiology/American Heart Association 2008 Guidelines for the Management of Adults with Congenital Heart Disease have simplified the process of deciding if and when to repair ASDs (*Figure 4*).[11] A significant ASD is gauged by the presence of right heart enlargement. If the right heart is enlarged without an alternative explanation, consideration should be made for repair, even in the absence of symptoms (Class I, Level of Evidence B recommendation).

At this time, only the secundum ASD has been successfully occluded through percutaneous methods (available devices are shown in *Figure 5*). All other types of ASD require surgical closure. Careful hemodynamics should be collected prior to repair to ensure that the PVR is not prohibitive for repair. Patients with PVR greater than two-thirds the systemic PVR or an absolute PVR >7 Wood's units should not undergo immediate repair, but may be eligible for medical therapy that targets PAH. Transient balloon occlusion or pulmonary vasodilator testing also may assist the timing of intervention.

Early repair of ASD appears to be most optimal. Closure after the age of 40 is associated with an increased incidence of arrhythmias (atrial fibrillation) compared with closure before age 40 (*Figure 6*). Epidemiologic evidence also suggests that long-term survival is worse with unrepaired defects (*Figure 7*). Age itself, however, should not exclude consideration of ASD repair. Occasionally, patients can present late in life with ASD-related symptoms when the left atrial pressure rises because of a stiff left ventricle and diastolic dysfunction (usually the result of long-standing hypertension or coronary artery disease).

Another type of ASD is the primum ASD, which involves the lower portion of the atrial septum and typically affects the ventricular septum as well (the so-called AV canal defect; *Videos 8, 9*). Both AV valves are structurally abnormal, and the mitral valve is typically cleft (*Video 10*). As a result of the anatomical position of the conduction bundles, a superior left axis usually is noted in primum ASD. Primum defects commonly are seen in patients with trisomy 21 (Down syndrome) and frequently present early in life because of their significant impact on cardiovascular physiology. This defect is only repairable surgically and ideally by a surgeon experienced in this repair.

A less common variation of ASD is the sinus venosus ASD, in which there is abnormal fusion of the SVC or IVC to the LA. This defect is almost always associated with partial anomalous return of the PVs (right superior or both right PVs draining into the SVC or RA). Because of its location, this defect can be missed on transthoracic echocardiography and usually requires either transesophageal echocardiogram (*Video 11*) or advanced radiographic imaging to make the diagnosis. The least common ASD, the CS septal defect, involves unroofing of the CS, which results in shunting from the LA to the RA. Commonly, a persistent left SVC or abnormal pulmonary venous drainage accompanies CS ASD.

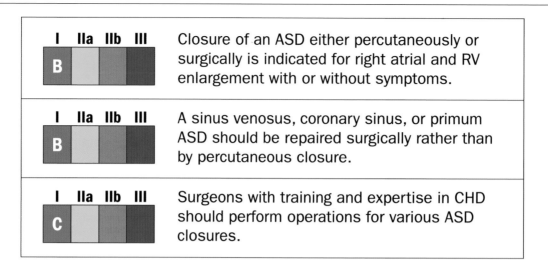

I	**IIa**	**IIb**	**III**	Closure of an ASD either percutaneously or surgically is indicated for right atrial and RV enlargement with or without symptoms.
	B			

I	**IIa**	**IIb**	**III**	A sinus venosus, coronary sinus, or primum ASD should be repaired surgically rather than by percutaneous closure.
	B			

I	**IIa**	**IIb**	**III**	Surgeons with training and expertise in CHD should perform operations for various ASD closures.
	C			

Figure 4

Guidelines Regarding Atrial Septal Defect Closure

ASD = atrial septal defect; CHD = congenital heart disease; RV = right ventricle.

Reproduced with permission from Warnes CA, Williams RG, Bashore TM, et al. ACC/AHA 2008 guidelines for the management of adults with congenital heart disease: a report of the American College of Cardiology/American Heart Association Task Force on Practice Guidelines (Writing Committee to Develop Guidelines on the Management of Adults With Congenital Heart Disease). Developed in Collaboration With the American Society of Echocardiography, Heart Rhythm Society, International Society for Adult Congenital Heart Disease, Society for Cardiovascular Angiography and Interventions, and Society of Thoracic Surgeons. J Am Coll Cardiol 2008;52:e143-263.

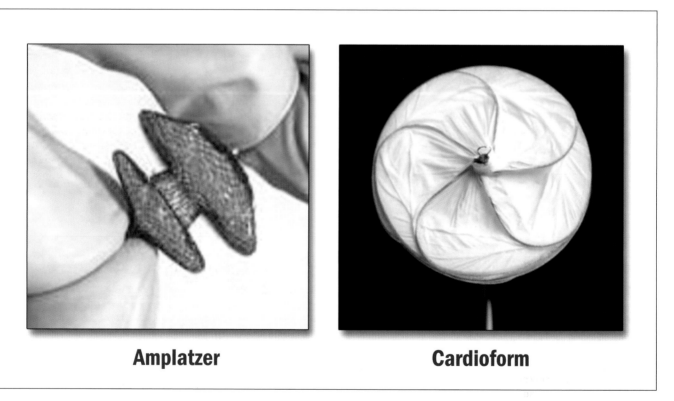

Amplatzer **Cardioform**

Figure 5

Currently Available Atrial Septal Defect Occluders

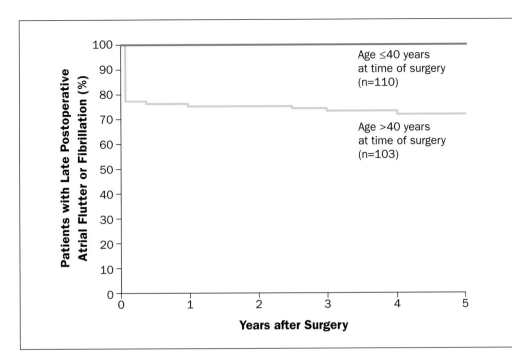

Figure 6

Atrial Fibrillation as Source of Morbidity Following Surgical Repair

Reproduced with permission from Gatzoulis MA, Freeman MA, Siu SC, Webb GD, Harris L. Atrial arrhythmia after surgical closure of atrial septal defects in adults. N Engl J Med 1999;340:839-46.

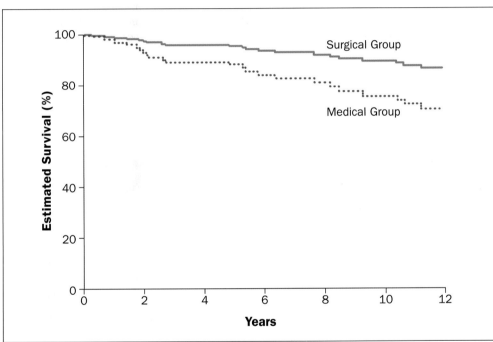

Figure 7

Medical Therapy Versus Surgery for Atrial Septal Defect

Reproduced with permission from Konstantinides S, Geibel A, Olschewski M, et al. A comparison of surgical and medical therapy for atrial septal defect in adults. N Engl J Med 1995;333:469-73.

 Video - not available for print.

Video 8

Atrioventricular Canal-type Defect on Apical 4-Chamber Echo View

The apical 4-chamber view shows dropout of both the ventricular septum (above) and atrial septum (below). The mitral (right of screen) and tricuspid valve (left of screen) appear at the same level. The lack of apical displacement of the tricuspid valve relative to the mitral valve is seen with atrioventricular canal-type defects.

 Video - not available for print.

Video 9

Close-up of Atrioventricular Canal-Type Defect on Apical 4-Chamber Echo View Using Color Doppler

Color Doppler demonstrates left-to-right shunting at both the atrial (below) and ventricular (above) levels. This is consistent with a balanced atrioventricular canal-type defect.

Video - not available for print.

Video 10

Cleft Anterior Leaflet of Mitral Valve on Parasternal Short-Axis Echo View

The parasternal short-axis view demonstrates a defect present in the middle of the anterior leaflet of the mitral valve consistent with a cleft. These are commonly seen with atrioventricular canal-type defects.

Video - not available for print.

Video 11

Sinus Venosus ASD on Bicaval TEE View with Color Doppler

Bicaval view on transesophageal echocardiogram which shows a large sinus venosus defect (on the right of the screen). The left atrium is on the top of the image and the right atrium on the bottom. An anomalous right upper pulmonary vein is usually present in such defects and is suggested in this image by the color flow just below the defect in the septum.

Key Points

- Significant ASDs lead to right heart enlargement, pulmonary hypertension, and atrial arrhythmias if unrepaired.

- Any patient with an ASD and otherwise unexplained right heart enlargement should be considered for ASD repair.

- Percutaneous closure is now the standard of care for most secundum ASDs. Only secundum ASD is amenable to percutaneous closure, and candidates should have adequate septal rims and normal pulmonary venous return.

- Patients with pulmonary hypertension should be carefully evaluated before closure of an ASD is attempted.

Partial Anomalous Pulmonary Venous Return

PAPVR should be suspected in any patient with evidence of unexplained right- sided volume overload. It is present in approximately 10% of secundum ASDs and nearly all patients with sinus venosus ASDs. Anomalous PVs include the left upper PV to the innominate vein (sometimes called a "vertical vein" because of its orientation), the right upper PV to the SVC or RA, or the right lower PV to the IVC (scimitar syndrome).

PAPVR can result in right ventricular volume overload and atrial arrhythmias and occasionally can lead to increased pulmonary pressures, particularly when more than one PV is anomalous. In cases where an ASD does not coexist, it is important to recognize that a bubble study will not assist in its detection (right-to-left shunting is not possible with this lesion). Surgical repair generally consists of diverting the PV flow back to the left atrium and can be accomplished with very low morbidity and mortality under the care of a capable surgeon.[12]

Key Points

- PAPVR is almost always present in patients with sinus venosus ASD.

- PAPVR in the absence of ASD will not cause a positive echo bubble study, but can result in right heart enlargement and pulmonary hypertension.

References

1. Gupta V, Tonelli A, Krasuski RA. Congenital heart disease and pulmonary hypertension. Heart Failure Clin 2012;8:427-45.

2. Krasuski RA. When and how to fix a 'hole in the heart': approach to ASD and PFO. Cleve Clin J Med 2007;74:137-47.

3. Hart SA, Krasuski RA. Incidence of asymptomatic patent foramen ovale according to age. Ann Intern Med 2009;150:431-2.

4. Meissner I, Khandheria BK, Heit JA, et al. Patent foramen ovale: innocent or guilty? Evidence from a prospective population-based study. J Am Coll Cardiol 2006;47:440-5.

5. Devendra G, Rane AA, Krasuski RA. Provoked exercise desaturation in patent foramen ovale and impact of percutaneous closure. J Am Coll Cardiol Cardiovasc Interv 2012;5:416-9.

6. Furlan AJ, Reisman M, Massaro J, et al., on behalf of the CLOSURE I Investigators. Closure or medical therapy for cryptogenic stroke with patent foramen ovale. N Engl J Med 2012;366:991-9.

7. Carroll JD, Saver JL, Thaler DE, et al., on behalf of the RESPECT Investigators. Closure of patent foramen ovale versus medical therapy after cryptogenic stroke. N Engl J Med 2013;368:1092-100.

8. Meier B, Kalesan B, Mattle H, et al., on behalf of the PC Trial Investigators. Percutaneous closure of patent foramen ovale in cryptogenic stroke. N Engl J Med 2013;368:1083-91.

9. Dowson A, Mullen MJ, Peatfield R, et al. Migraine Intervention With STARFlex Technology (MIST) trial: a prospective, multicenter, double-blind, sham-controlled trial to evaluate the effectiveness of patent foramen ovale closure with STARFlex septal repair implant to resolve refractory migraine headache. Circulation 2008;117:1397-404.

10. Mas JL, Arquizan C, Lamy C, et al., on behalf of the Patent Foramen Ovale and Atrial Septal Aneurysm Study Group. Recurrent cerebrovascular events associated with patent foramen ovale, atrial septal aneurysm, or both. N Engl J Med 2001;345:1740-6.

11. Warnes CA, Williams RG, Bashore TM, et al. ACC/AHA 2008 guidelines for the management of adults with congenital heart disease: a report of the American College of Cardiology/American Heart Association Task Force on Practice Guidelines (Writing Committee to Develop Guidelines on the Management of Adults With Congenital Heart Disease). Developed in Collaboration With the American Society of Echocardiography, Heart Rhythm Society, International Society for Adult Congenital Heart Disease, Society for Cardiovascular Angiography and Interventions, and Society of Thoracic Surgeons. J Am Coll Cardiol 2008;52:e143-263.

12. Majdalany DS, Phillips SD, Dearani JA, Connolly HM, Warnes CA. Isolated partial anomalous pulmonary venous connections in adults: twenty-year experience. Congenit Heart Dis 2010;5:537-45.

Congenital Heart Disease

Left Ventricular Outflow Tract Lesions

Introduction

Left ventricular outflow tract (LVOT) lesions typically refer to obstructive lesions below, at, or above the level of the aortic valve, including the subvalvular region, valvular aortic lesions, and supravalvular AS (including CoA). This module reviews the anatomy and physiology, clinical examination findings, diagnostic testing, and management for each of these lesions.

Subaortic Stenosis

Definition: Anatomy and Physiology

Subaortic stenosis refers to a discrete fibrous ring or a fibromuscular narrowing, and is distinctly different from hypertrophic cardiomyopathy-associated LVOT obstruction. Subaortic stenosis is often associated with other congenital heart abnormalities, such as ventricular septal defect (VSD), atrioventricular canal defect (AV Canal), or other conotruncal abnormalities.[1,2] If associated with these defects, subaortic stenosis typically forms/progresses after patch closure of the VSD (*Figure 1*).

Subaortic stenosis is usually progressive, and can lead to LV hypertension/hypertrophy and failure, aortic valve damage with resultant aortic insufficiency, higher risk for infective endocarditis, and sudden cardiac death.[3]

Clinical Exam and Associated Lesions

The physical exam of a patient with subaortic stenosis is characterized by a crescendo-decrescendo harsh systolic murmur in varying degrees of intensity. This murmur is best heard along the left sternal boarder and apex, and radiates throughout the precordium. Additionally, if there is associated aortic insufficiency secondary to aortic valve injury, there may be an early diastolic murmur along the left sternal boarder.

Subaortic stenosis can be associated with other congenital heart defects, such as VSD, AV Canal defect, conotruncal abnormalities, or may develop after patch closure of a perimembranous or misaligned VSD/AV Canal defect.[4]

Diagnostic Testing

Lifelong care is recommended for patients with subaortic stenosis, with a cardiologist who has expertise in adult congenital heart disease (ACHD). Asymptomatic patients with a mean gradient ≥30 mm Hg and no LV hypertrophy are recommended to have a yearly evaluation to monitor increasing obstruction, change in aortic valve insufficiency, or the development of LV hypertrophy, and any reduction in the LV systolic and/or diastolic function (*Figure 2*).

In patients for whom the criteria for intervention is equivocal, exercise stress testing may be performed to determine exercise capacity and symptoms, and an electrocardiogram (ECG) may be performed to determine changes or arrhythmias. Additionally, stress echocardiography helps to define the increase in the gradient with exercise.[3]

Amanda S. Green, FNP-C
This author has nothing to disclose.

John F. Rhodes Jr, MD, FACC
Consultant Fees/Honoraria: W.L. Gore & Associates.

Learner Objectives

Upon completion of this module, the reader will be able to:

1. Discuss surgical indications for patients with subvalvular aortic stenosis (AS).
2. Discuss surgical/transcatheter indications for patients with valvular AS.
3. Recognize the importance of complete evaluation of the ascending aorta in evaluation for supravalvular AS.
4. Describe the classic physical exam and imaging findings in patients with unrepaired coarctation of the aorta (CoA).

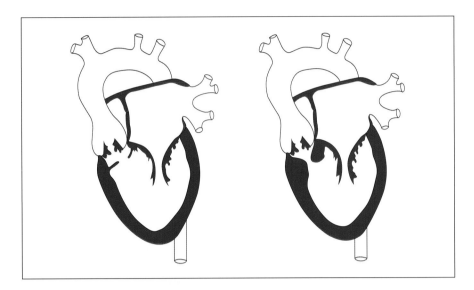

Figure 1
Schematic of the Types of Subaortic Stenosis

Management of Subaortic Stenosis

Management of the subaortic membrane is largely surgical. In asymptomatic patients, surgery is recommended for a peak gradient ≥50 mm Hg and/or mean gradient ≥30 mm Hg by echocardiography. If there is progressive aortic insufficiency and an LV end-systolic dimension of >50 mm or an LV ejection fraction <50%, surgical resection of the subaortic obstruction is recommended, even if the gradients are less than these levels. Surgical recommendations are outlined in *Table 1*.[3]

Key Point
• Subaortic stenosis is often a progressive lesion. This can lead to damage of the aortic valve, typically manifested by aortic insufficiency and subsequent LV dysfunction.

Valvular Aortic Stenosis (Noncalcific Aortic Valve Stenosis)

Definition: Anatomy and Physiology

Valvular AS can often be attributed to a bicuspid aortic valve, or less commonly, a unicuspid aortic valve. The bicuspid aortic valve is the most common congenital heart defect, and is seen in as many as 1-2% of the general population.[1] LVOT occurs at the level of the aortic valve itself. In pediatric populations, this occurs most commonly with stenotic and/or abnormal aortic valve apparatus.

With aging, there is a higher rate of calcification of the valve, thus creating obstruction of the aortic valve on both normal trileaflet valves, and an accelerated process of calcification of bicuspid valves (*Figure 3*). This lesion can occur as a unique finding or as a part of a constellation of other congenital heart abnormalities. CoA, mitral valve abnormalities, septal defects, and other conotruncal anomalies may also be present.[4]

The bicuspid valve commissural fusion is variable. In a retrospective review of 1,135 patients with a bicuspid aortic valve, the most common fusion was between the right and left coronary commissures (70%). Moderate or greater aortic stenosis was observed in patients with fusion of the right and noncoronary cusps (p ≤ 0.001). The majority of patients with bicuspid aortic valve and CoA had fusion of the right and left coronary commissures (89%), with lesser degrees of stenosis or insufficiency.[5]

Clinical Examination and Associated Lesions

The physical examination of a patient with AS may reveal a valve "click" (if the valve is mobile), and varying degrees of a systolic murmur associated with the AS. This murmur is best heard along the right sternal boarder, and typically radiates into the suprasternal notch and carotid arteries. A thrill can often be felt in the suprasternal notch. As the degree of AS worsens, the murmur may peak later in systole. Additionally, younger patients with worsening AS often have a delayed carotid upstroke.

Although bicuspid aortic valve/aortic valve abnormalities can be a singular occurrence, they can also be associated with other abnormalities such as subaortic obstruction, parachute (or other) mitral valve abnormalities, VSD, patent ductus arteriosus, CoA, or varying degrees of associated aortic arch hypoplasia. A bicuspid aortic valve is commonly associated with a left dominant coronary artery system. A bicuspid aortic valve can also be associated with progressive dilation or aneurysm of the aortic root and/or ascending aorta in 50% of the population.[4]

Associated Syndromes

The Turner syndrome is associated with aortic valve stenosis. Additionally, when multiple left-sided obstructive lesions occur together, this is classified as Shone's syndrome.[4]

Diagnostic Testing

Lifelong care is recommended for patients with aortic valve disease. Evaluation with echocardiography and ECG is recommended as routine testing for most patients at varying intervals based on their clinical findings. Each patient should have some type of aortic arch imaging (computed tomography [CT] or magnetic resonance [MRI]) at some stage to exclude an ascending aneurysm.

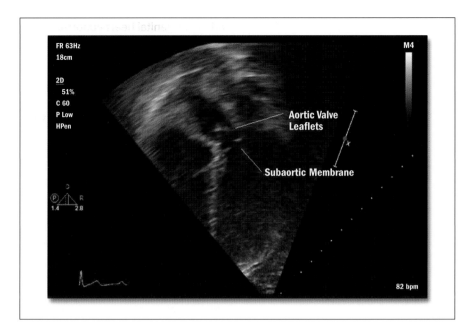

Figure 2
Echocardiographic Image of Membranous Subaortic Stenosis

○ A peak instantaneous gradient of >50 mm Hg or a mean gradient
of 30 mm Hg on Doppler echocardiography.

○ Progressive aortic regurgitation and a left ventricular end-systolic
dimension of >50 mm or a left ventricular ejection fraction <55%.

Table 1
Class I Recommendations for Surgical Intervention in Adults With Isolated Subaortic Stenosis

Modified from Warnes CA, Williams RG, Bashore TM, et al. ACC/AHA 2008 guidelines for the management of adults with congenital heart disease: executive summary: a report of the American College of Cardiology/American Heart Association Task Force on Practice Guidelines (writing committee to develop guidelines for the management of adults with congenital heart disease). J Am Coll Cardiol 2008;52:e143-263.

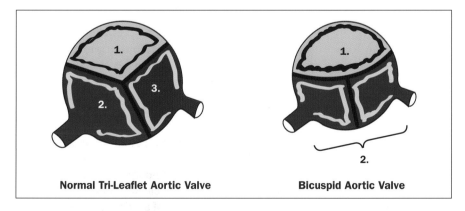

Normal Tri-Leaflet Aortic Valve　　　　**Bicuspid Aortic Valve**

Figure 3
Schematic of a Bicuspid Valve

Asymptomatic teens and young adults with a mean gradient ≥30 mm Hg and peak gradient ≥50 mm Hg are recommended to have a yearly ECG evaluation. Patients with a mean gradient <30 mm Hg and a peak gradient <50 mm Hg are recommended to have echocardiography or Doppler imaging and ECG follow-up every 2 years.

Echocardiography is also recommended to assess changes in patients with known AS who become pregnant.[3] Cardiac catheterization is recommended if noninvasive testing is inconclusive or inconsistent with the patient's clinical symptomatology.[3]

Management of Valvular Aortic Stenosis
Management strategies for progressive AS typically include cardiac catheterization or surgical management. *Table 2* summarizes recommendations from the 2008 American College of Cardiology/ American Heart Associaton Guidelines for the Management of Adults with Congenital Heart Disease.

In general, AS without insufficiency in teens and young adults can be managed in the catheterization laboratory with balloon aortic valvuloplasty. Surgical intervention is more commonly seen in patients with aortic insufficiency or in the older adult population where calcific valves are common.[3]

Supravalvular Aortic Stenosis

Definition: Anatomy and Physiology
Supravalvular AS refers to an hourglass appearance of the supravalvular aortic region, a discrete membrane in the supravalvular region, or diffuse tubular hypoplasia of the entire ascending aorta (*Figure 4*).

Supravalvular AS is rare, and is often associated with Williams syndrome, which frequently occurs with other associated left heart lesions, including peripheral pulmonary artery stenosis (30%), CoA (15%), renal artery stenosis (5%), and ostial coronary artery

Class I Recommendations for Catheter Interventions for Adults with Valvular Aortic Stenosis

- In young adults without significantly calcified aortic valves and no aortic insufficiency, balloon aortic valvuloplasty is indicated in the following patients:
  - Patients with symptoms of angina, syncope, dyspnea on exertion, and peak-to-peak gradients at catheterization of >50 mm Hg (Level of Evidence C).
  - Asymptomatic patients who demonstrate ST- or T-wave abnormalities in the left precordial leads on electrocardiogram at rest or with exercise and a peak-to-peak gradient in the catheterization laboratory >60 mm Hg.

Class I Recommendations for Surgical Aortic Valve Repair/Replacement and Aortic Root Replacement

- Aortic valvuloplasty, AVR, or Ross repair is indicated in patients with severe AS or chronic severe AR while they undergo coronary artery bypass grafting surgery on the aorta, or surgery on other heart valves (Level of Evidence C).
- AVR is indicated for patients with severe AS and LV dysfunction (LVEF<50%) (Level of Evidence C).
- AVR is indicated in adolescents or young adults with severe AR who have:
  - Development of symptoms (Level of Evidence C).
  - Development of persistent LV dysfunction (LVEF <50%) or progressive LV dilation (LV end-diastolic diameter 4 standard deviations above normal) (Level of Evidence C).
- Surgery to repair or replace the ascending aorta in a patient with a bicuspid aortic valve is recommended when the ascending aorta diameter is ≥5.0 cm or when there is progressive dilation at a rate ≥5 mm per year (Level of Evidence B).

Table 2

Management of Catheterization Versus Surgical Intervention in Valvular Stenosis

AR = aortic regurgitation; AS = aortic stenosis; AVR = aortic valve replacement; EF = ejection fraction; LV = left ventricular.

Modified from Warnes CA, Williams RG, Bashore TM, et al. ACC/AHA 2008 guidelines for the management of adults with congenital heart disease: executive summary: a report of the American College of Cardiology/American Heart Association Task Force on Practice Guidelines (writing committee to develop guidelines for the management of adults with congenital heart disease). J Am Coll Cardiol 2008;52:e143-263.

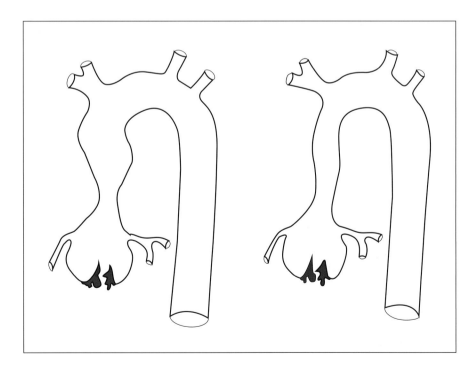

Figure 4

Schematic of Supravalvular Aortic Stenosis

stenosis (occurring as a result of the supravalvular aortic obstruction).[4] Of the patients with Williams syndrome, 85% have cardiovascular anomalies, with 71% having supravalvular AS.[4]

The physiology of supravalvular AS is similar to the physiology in valvular AS, except that the coronary arteries are on the high-pressure side of the lesion. The coronary artery ostium occasionally can become obstructed as a result of the supravalvular AS, thus resulting in the possibility of sudden cardiac death or coronary artery underperfusion relative to myocardial demands.[1,4]

Clinical Examination and Associated Lesions

On physical examination, there may be the presence of a harsh systolic murmur, heard over the base of the heart with radiation to the suprasternal notch and carotids. Depending on the degree of stenosis, there may

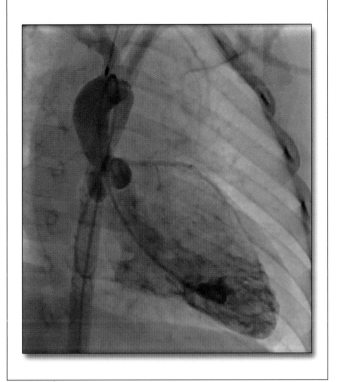

Figure 5

Supravalvular Aortic Stenosis Catheterization Angiogram in a Patient With Williams Syndrome

also be a thrill present in either or both the sternal boarder locations or at the suprasternal notch and carotids. Patients with Williams syndrome also may have classic facial "elfin" features, "cocktail" personalities, mental retardation, and small stature.[4]

Diagnostic Testing

If the supravalvular AS is severe, there may be LV hypertrophy present on the ECG. The chest X-ray often does not add much value in the diagnosis, unless there is cardiomegaly.

An echocardiogram is the most common modality for diagnosis, given that it provides a 2-D image of the LVOT and supravalvular aortic area. Doppler imaging can be used to estimate the pressure gradient across this area, and provide imaging of the brachiocephalic vessels and the remainder of the aorta to rule out coarctation.

Cardiac MRI is an excellent modality to provide anatomic information about the LV size, dimensions of the LVOT, area of supravalvular stenosis, presence of other brachiocephalic artery stenosis, CoA, degree of any aortic regurgitation, and renal artery stenosis. The MRI can also provide information about the proximal coronary arteries, and late gadolinium enhancement can evaluate for ventricular scar.

Cardiac catheterization can also be used as a diagnostic tool when there is a need for direct measurement of the hemodynamic gradients to determine the timing or need for surgical repair (*Figure 5*).

- ○ Operative intervention should be performed for patients with supravalvular AS (discrete or diffuse) with symptoms, such as angina, dyspnea, or syncope, and/or a mean gradient >50 mm Hg or peak gradient by echocardiography Doppler >70 mm Hg (Level of Evidence B).

- ○ Surgical repair is recommended for adults with lesser degrees of supravalvular LVOT obstruction and the following indications:
  - Symptoms: angina, dyspnea, or syncope (Level of Evidence B).
  - LV Hypertrophy (Level of Evidence C).
  - Desire for greater degrees of exercise or a planned pregnancy (Level of Evidence C).
  - LV systolic dysfunction (Level of Evidence C).

- ○ Interventions for coronary artery obstruction in patients with supravalvular AS should be performed in ACHD centers with demonstrated expertise in the interventional management of such patients (Level of Evidence C).

Table 3

Class I Recommendations for Intervention in Supravalvular Aortic Stenosis

ACHD = adult congenital heart disease; AS = aortic stenosis; LVOT = left ventricular outflow tract.

Modified from Warnes CA, Williams RG, Bashore TM, et al. ACC/AHA 2008 guidelines for the management of adults with congenital heart disease: executive summary: a report of the American College of Cardiology/American Heart Association Task Force on Practice Guidelines (writing committee to develop guidelines for the management of adults with congenital heart disease). J Am Coll Cardiol 2008;52:e143-263.

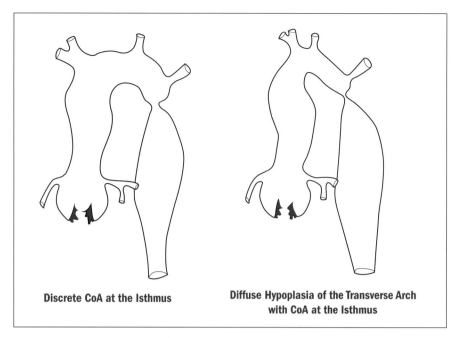

Figure 6

Diagram of Coarctation of the Aorta

CoA = coarctation of the aorta.

Discrete CoA at the Isthmus

Diffuse Hypoplasia of the Transverse Arch with CoA at the Isthmus

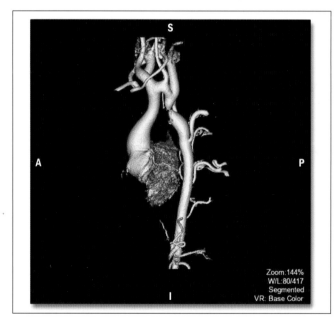

S

A   P

Zoom:144%
W/L:80/417
Segmented
VR: Base Color

I

Figure 7

Computed Tomography Angiogram of Native Coarctation of the Aorta With Transverse Aortic Arch Hypoplasia

Management of Supravalvular Aortic Stenosis

Surgical management should be considered when the mean gradient is ≥50 mm Hg or the peak gradient is ≥70 mm Hg by echocardiography. A lesser degree of obstruction warrants intervention if clinical symptoms, including angina, dyspnea, or syncope, emerge (*Table 3*).

Patients should have yearly follow-up at a regional center for ACHD, irrespective of their surgical status. Patients with Williams syndrome should have long-term psychosocial assessment and oversight, and they may even need legal guardianship.[3]

Coarctation of the Aorta

Definition: Anatomy and Physiology

CoA is usually classified by a discrete narrowing of the aorta in the proximal descending aorta (at the isthmus). However, CoA also can involve hypoplasia of the transverse aortic arch. The precise cause of CoA is not known, but it is believed to be related to either an abnormal flow pattern or is secondary to the involvement of ductal tissue in the normal aortic wall (*Figure 6*).

In patients whose ductal tissue extends into the normal aorta, the closure of the ductus arteriosus leads to constriction of the normal aortic segment and subsequent CoA itself. In patients with abnormal flow patterns, there is diminished blood flow through the ascending aorta in utero, and this may be secondary to an abnormality in the left heart, such as mitral valve disease (stenosis/ hypoplasia), VSD, or subaortic obstruction.[6,7]

The reverse is also true. With right heart outflow obstructive lesions, where there is decreased flow through the pulmonary arteries and increased flow through the aortic arch (such as pulmonary atresia or tetralogy of Fallot), CoA is rarely seen.[7]

The timing of symptoms related to CoA varies. As neonatal diagnostic technology has improved, there are fewer patients with CoA who remain undiagnosed and present later in life. Symptoms include hypertension, headaches, or claudication of the lower extremities.[7]

Clinical Examination and Associated Lesions

CoA can be associated with bicuspid aortic valve, particularly bicuspid valve with fusion of the left and right intracoronary commissures in 89% of patients.[5] CoA also has associations with the Turner and Williams syndromes.[7]

The physical examination for CoA notes a systolic or continuous murmur at the left interscapular region and base of the heart, with the murmur louder at the former, radiating posteriorly along the spine. If collateral arteries are present around the coarctation, then a continuous nature of the murmur, or extension of the murmur

Class I Recommendations for Interventional and Surgical Treatment of Coarctation of the Aorta in Adults

- Intervention for CoA is recommended in the following circumstances:
  - Peak-to-peak coarctation gradient ≥20 mm Hg (Level of Evidence C).
  - Peak-to-peak coarctation gradient <20 mm Hg in the presence of anatomic imaging evidence of significant coarctation with radiological evidence of significant collateral flow (Level of Evidence C).
- Choice of percutaneous catheter intervention versus surgical repair of native discrete coarctation should be determined by consultation with a team of ACHD cardiologists, interventionalists, and surgeons at an ACHD center (Level of Evidence C).
- Percutaneous catheter intervention is indicated for recurrent, discrete coarctation and a peak-to-peak gradient of at least 20 mm Hg (Level of Evidence B).
- Surgeons with training and expertise in ACHD should perform operations for previously repaired coarctation and the following indications:
  - Long recoarctation segment (Level of Evidence B).
  - Concomitant hypoplasia of the aortic arch (Level of Evidence B).

Table 4

Class I Recommendations for Interventional and Surgical Treatment of Coarctation of the Aorta in Adults

ACHD = adult congenital heart disease; CoA = coarctation of the aorta.

Modified from Warnes CA, Williams RG, Bashore TM, et al. ACC/AHA 2008 guidelines for the management of adults with congenital heart disease: executive summary: a report of the American College of Cardiology/American Heart Association Task Force on Practice Guidelines (writing committee to develop guidelines for the management of adults with congenital heart disease). J Am Coll Cardiol 2008;52:e143-263.

into diastole, may be audible, and is secondary to the continuation of flow into the descending aorta.

Additional physical examination findings may include an aortic valve ejection click if the valve is mobile, upper extremity hypertension, and a delay between the upper extremity and femoral pulsations. The femoral pulses are often weak, if at all palpable.

CoA is also associated with cerebral aneurysms, which have been found as frequently as up to 10% of adults.[8] Complete understanding of this is not known, but is thought to be a sequela of long-standing upper extremity hypertension or an inherited pathogenic factor, which is ultimately responsible for both the coarctation and the berry aneurysm.[8]

Diagnostic Testing

The simplest of diagnostic tests is measuring four extremity blood pressures, with the patient in the supine position. Care should be taken to use an appropriately sized blood pressure cuff to ensure accuracy in the measured blood pressures. Patients who have CoA will have diminished blood pressure in their lower extremities.

In the adult population, determining whether this diminished blood pressure is secondary to CoA versus peripheral arterial disease can be difficult. A lower extremity blood pressure ≥20 mm Hg less than the upper extremity blood pressure (right arm is preferable) is

considered significant. Recall that the lower extremity systolic blood pressure should be higher than in the upper extremity due to reflected waveforms from the peripheral resistance.

The ECG may demonstrate LV hypertrophy, depending on the degree of upper body hypertension. Transthoracic echocardiography can provide imaging of the aortic arch and the isthmus. However, in adults, it can be difficult to fully evaluate this because of the poor patient echocardiographic windows. Yet, the echocardiogram may provide additional clues, such as LV hypertrophy, and evaluation of the abdominal aortic area. Doppler imaging may demonstrate blunting or continuation of flow into diastole.

Additional imaging, such as cardiac MRI or CT, can be used to evaluate the aortic arch. This provides comprehensive images of the aortic arch that can be made into 3-D images, which are very important in the planning and management of CoA (*Figure 7*).

Key Point

- Classic examination findings of CoA are: systemic hypertension, brachial-femoral pulse delay, and decreased pulsatility with blunting of the abdominal aortic Doppler pattern. A gradient of 20 mm Hg across the lesion is considered to be significant.

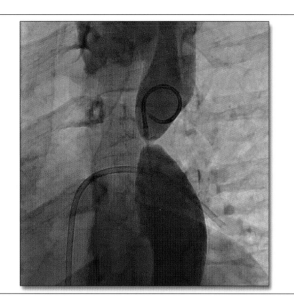

Figure 8

Cardiac Catheterization Image Showing Severe Native Coarctation of the Aorta With Near Interruption and Hypoplasia of the Transverse Arch

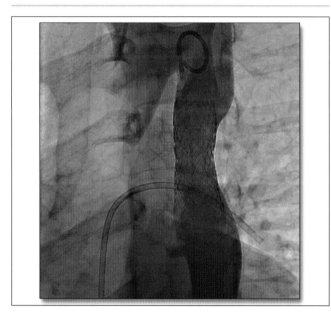

Figure 9

Cardiac Catheterization Image Showing Native Coarctation of the Aorta Following Stent Angioplasty of the Aorta at the Isthmus

Management of Coarctation of the Aorta

Medical management should be considered when there is upper extremity hypertension, using beta-blockers, angiotensin-converting enzyme inhibitors, or angiotensin-receptor blockers. The choice of medication class can be determined in part by the presence of aortic root dilation or aortic insufficiency.

An indication for intervention is a coarctation peak-to-peak gradient of 20 mm Hg across the lesion. Interventional versus surgical management of native discrete CoA (*Table 4*) should be determined by a team of ACHD surgeons, interventionalists, and cardiologists at an ACHD center. For recurrent arch obstruction, transcatheter intervention is indicated for discrete recurrent coarctation and a peak-to-peak gradient ≥20 mm Hg. Surgical repair of recurrent coarctation is indicated when there is a long-segment coarctation and/or hypoplasia of the transverse aortic arch[3] (*Figures 8, 9*).

Lifelong yearly follow-up with an ACHD center, along with close monitoring of blood pressure for hypertension, is recommended for patients with both repaired and unrepaired CoA. In patients with repaired CoA, by either surgical or catheter technique, diagnostic testing should include MRI or CT evaluation of the aorta at least every 5 years. Exercise testing performed at intervals determined by the ACHD cardiologist may also be used to help determine if recurrent obstruction is a concern, and to help determine the timing of reintervention.

Key Point

- Patients who have had transcatheter or surgical repair of CoA should have routine follow-up cardiac MRI or CT every 5 years.

References

1. Edwards JE. Pathophysiology of left ventricular outflow tract obstruction. Circulation 1965;31:586-99.

2. Maron BJ, Redwood DR, Roberts WC, Henry WL, Morrow AG, Epstein SE. Tunnel subaortic stenosis: left ventricular outflow tract obstruction produced by fibromuscular tubular narrowing. Circulation 1976;54:404-16.

3. Warnes CA, Williams RG, Bashore TM, et al. ACC/AHA 2008 guidelines for the management of adults with congenital heart disease: executive summary: a report of the American College of Cardiology/American Heart Association Task Force on Practice Guidelines (writing committee to develop guidelines for the management of adults with congenital heart disease). J Am Coll Cardiol 2008;52:e143-263.

4. Keane JF, Fyler DC. Aortic outflow obstructions. In: Keane JF, Fyler DC, Lock JE, eds. Nadas' Pediatric Cardiology. 2nd ed. Philadelphia: Saunders; 2006:581-601.

5. Fernandes SM, Sanders SP, Khairy P, et al. Morphology of bicuspid aortic valve in children and adolescents. J Am Coll Cardiol 2004;44:1648-51.

6. Campbell M. Natural history of coarctation of the aorta. Br Heart J 1970;32:633-40.

7. Keane JF, Fyler DC. Coarctation of the aorta. In: Keane JF, Fyler DC, Lock JE, eds. Nadas' Pediatric Cardiology. 2nd ed. Philadelphia: Saunders; 2006:627-44.

8. Curtis SL, Bradley M, Wilde P, et al. Results of screening for intracranial aneurysm in patients with coarctation of the aorta. AJNR Am J Neuroradiol 2012;33:1182-6.

Right Ventricular Outflow Tract Lesions and Complex Lesions

Pulmonary Valve Stenosis

Definition: Anatomy and Physiology

Congenital valvular pulmonary stenosis (PS) is a common anomaly with a variable clinical presentation. Many children with milder forms of PS may be asymptomatic, and the condition may be discovered during their adult years. Adults with PS most often have a thickened valve with commissural fusion or a bicuspid valve. Poststenotic dilation of the main and branch pulmonary arteries (PAs) is common, as is mild pulmonary regurgitation (PR). Calcification of the valve is uncommon, even in older patients. In a study of 325 patients with congenital PS, doming was present in 31%, leaflet thickening in 24%, and calcification in 1-2%.

Clinical Exam and Associated Lesions

The clinical examination findings of congenital PS reflect a hypertrophied, noncompliant right ventricle (RV) and abnormal valve morphology. This includes a prominent jugular A wave, a RV lift, a soft and delayed second heart sound as a result of prolonged ejection time, and a crescendo-decrescendo systolic ejection murmur, which lengthens and peaks later in systole with increasing obstruction. The loudness of the classic "systolic ejection click" is dependent on having a stiff valve and adequate excursion of the valve to create the click sound. In congenital PS, the RV end-diastolic pressure is elevated while the PA pressure is normal, and the atrial kick into the RV increases the pressure to prematurely open the pulmonary valve before systole. With inspiration, the right heart pressure further increases and the valve opens even more prematurely, which further reduces the valve excursion in systole and the intensity of the click is lessened.

Congenital PS is often an isolated congenital heart lesion; however, it may be associated with infundibular stenosis, supravalvular or branch PA stenosis, or atrial septal defect (ASD). Abnormalities of the pulmonary valve may be present in adults with certain genetic syndromes, such as Noonan syndrome, Williams syndrome, Trisomy 13-15 and 18, and congenital rubella syndrome.[1] The frequency of PS in Noonan syndrome is approximately 25%, with 7% of these cases demonstrating a dysplastic pulmonary valve that may not be responsive to balloon angioplasty.

Diagnostic Testing

Transthoracic echocardiography (TTE) is the imaging modality of choice for evaluation of congenital PS. Leaflet thickening enhances visualization of the valve, and PA poststenotic dilation is a helpful clue in previously unsuspected valvular pathology. Classic valvular stenosis causes systolic doming of the leaflets (*Figure 1*). Pulsed wave Doppler demonstrates an increase in systolic velocity that begins at the valvular level, and continuous wave Doppler allows estimation of the peak and mean transvalvular gradient.

Anne Marie Valente, MD, FACC
This author has nothing to disclose.

Learner Objectives

Upon completion of this module, the reader will be able to:

1. Describe the physical examination findings of a patient with valvular pulmonary stenosis (PS).
2. Recognize the imaging appearance of double-chamber right ventricle (DCRV).
3. Evaluate for long-term sequelae in adults with repaired tetralogy of Fallot (TOF).
4. Discuss the long-term sequelae in adults with surgically repaired complete transposition of the great arteries (TGA).
5. Consider the importance of tricuspid regurgitation (systemic atrioventricular [AV] valve regurgitation) in patients with physiologically corrected TGA.
6. Recognize the heterogeneity of double outlet RV (DORV) and describe the several types of physiology that may be present.
7. Discuss the anatomy and physiology of Ebstein anomaly and recognize the arrhythmias that are associated with Ebstein anomaly.

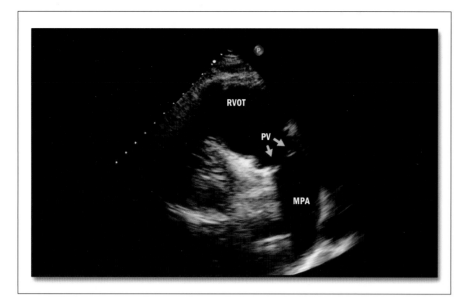

Figure 1

Parasternal Long-Axis Echocardiographic View of the Right Ventricular Outflow Tract in a Patient With Valvular Pulmonary Stenosis

The valve leaflets are thickened and dome into the pulmonary artery during systole (arrows). There is a poststenotic dilation of the main pulmonary artery.

MPA = main pulmonary artery; PV = pulmonary valve; RVOT = right ventricular outflow tract.

Reproduced with permission from Valente AM, King ME. Echocardiographic evaluation of the adult congenital heart disease patient with no prior cardiac procedures. In: Otto C, ed. The Practice of Clinical Echocardiography. 4th ed. Philadelphia: Elsevier Saunders; 2012.

Color flow mapping distinctly delineates the turbulent jet of high-velocity flow into the main PA. Accurate peak Doppler flow velocities may be difficult to obtain from the parasternal approach as a result of the horizontal substernal course of the right ventricular outflow tract (RVOT) and a more accurate peak systolic velocity may be sampled from the apical or subxiphoid approach. Long-standing valvular obstruction leads to significant RV hypertrophy, including the infundibular portion of the ventricle. Dynamic infundibular obstruction contributes to the increasing valvular gradient over time. Doppler flow patterns sampled within the infundibulum typically demonstrate dagger-shaped, late-peaking systolic envelope suggestive of dynamic obstruction.

Management

The asymptomatic adult with mild PS requires no intervention. The second natural history study of congenital heart defects reported that patients with mild PS (peak gradient <25 mm Hg) have less than a 5% chance of requiring intervention in adulthood.

○ Balloon valvotomy is recommended for asymptomatic patients with a domed pulmonary valve and a peak instantaneous Doppler gradient >60 mm Hg or a mean Doppler gradient >40 mm Hg (in association with less than moderate pulmonary regurgitation).

○ Balloon valvotomy is recommended for symptomatic patients with a domed pulmonary valve and a peak instantaneous Doppler gradient >50 mm Hg or a mean Doppler gradient >30 mm Hg (in association with less than moderate pulmonary regurgitation).

○ Surgical therapy is recommended for patients with severe PS and an associated hypoplastic pulmonary annulus, severe pulmonary regurgitation, subvalvular PS, or supravalvular PS. Surgery is also preferred for most dysplastic pulmonary valves, and when there is associated severe TR or the need for a surgical Maze procedure.

Table 1

Class I Recommendations for Intervention in Adults With Congenital Pulmonary Stenosis

PS = pulmonary stenosis; TR = tricuspid regurgitation.

Modified from Warnes CA, Williams RG, Bashore TM, et al. ACC/AHA 2008 guidelines for the management of adults with congenital heart disease: a report of the American College of Cardiology/American Heart Association Task Force on Practice Guidelines (Writing Committee to Develop Guidelines on the Management of Adults With Congenital Heart Disease). Developed in Collaboration With the American Society of Echocardiography, Heart Rhythm Society, International Society for Adult Congenital Heart Disease, Society for Cardiovascular Angiography and Interventions, and Society of Thoracic Surgeons. J Am Coll Cardiol 2008;52:e143-263.

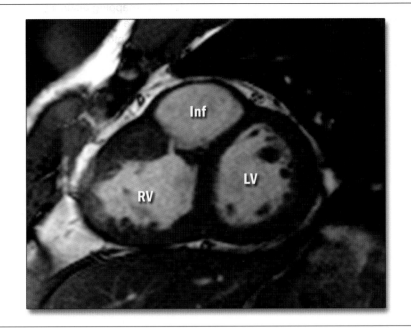

Figure 2

Cine Magnetic Resonance Image in the Short-Axis Plane Demonstrating a Double-Chamber Right Ventricle

There is muscular narrowing at the proximal os infundibulum, which is the junction of the right ventricular sinus and the infundibulum. The obstruction separates the RV into high- and low-pressure chambers and may be associated with a membranous ventricular septal defect.

Inf = infundibulum; LV = left ventricle; RV = right ventricle.

Reproduced with permission from Valente AM, Powell AJ. Clinical applications of cardiovascular magnetic resonance in congenital heart disease. Magn Reson Imaging Clin N Am 2007;15:565-77.

Those with moderate degrees of stenosis (peak gradient of 25-50 mm Hg) have only a 20% likelihood of requiring an intervention later in life.

Table 1 summarizes the American College of Cardiology/American Heart Association (ACC/AHA) 2008 Guidelines for the Management of Adults With Congenital Heart Disease Class I recommendations for intervention in adults with PS.[2] Balloon valvuloplasty is the treatment of choice for isolated congenital PS; it is safe and provides good long-term results.[3] Factors contributing to a poor response to balloon dilation include a small pulmonary valve annulus, markedly thickened, and significant infundibular hypertrophy. Regression of hypertrophy does occur in a large percentage of patients after removal of the valvular component of obstruction and does not constitute an absolute contraindication to balloon valvuloplasty.

Key Points

- The pulmonary systolic ejection click becomes softer with inspiration as a result of increased RV pressure and premature opening of the pulmonary valve, with reduced valve excursion during systole.

- Twenty-five percent of patients with Noonan's syndrome have PS and this is often a dysplastic pulmonary valve.

- Asymptomatic adults with congenital PS and a peak systolic gradient of <25 mm Hg rarely require intervention. A significant mean gradient in an asymptomatic adult is considered to be 40 mm Hg.

Double-Chamber Right Ventricle

Definition: Anatomy and Physiology
DCRV is characterized by obstruction within the RV caused by marked hypertrophy of muscle bundles within the RVOT. The moderator band may be displaced, creating narrowing of the proximal portion of the os infundibulum. The RV is divided into a high-pressure proximal sinus chamber and a low-pressure distal infundibular chamber. A perimembranous ventricular septal defect (VSD) is common. The location of the VSD determines the clinical features of this lesion. If the VSD is located proximal to the obstructing muscle bundles, pulmonary blood flow usually is decreased and right-to-left shunting exists across the VSD, which may cause cyanosis. Adults with DCRV may have had a VSD close earlier in life, and subaortic stenosis may be present. There is a progressive increase in the RVOT gradient, ranging from 3.3 to 11.1 mm Hg per year in one series.[4]

Clinical Exam
The diagnosis of DCRV may be missed if the systolic murmur heard on exam is attributed solely to a restrictive VSD. The systolic ejection murmur is classically located at the mid-left sternal border and may be accompanied by a thrill and a RV heave in the setting of significant obstruction. The second heart sound is usually normal in intensity and splitting, as the pulmonary valve is not affected in this condition.

Diagnostic Testing
The electrocardiogram findings in this condition can vary from normal to RV hypertrophy and right axis deviation. An upright T wave in lead V_3R is a clue to this diagnosis because this is not a typical finding in patients with a VSD or TOF. TTE reveals the subvalvular obstruction; however, acoustic windows in adults may be challenging.

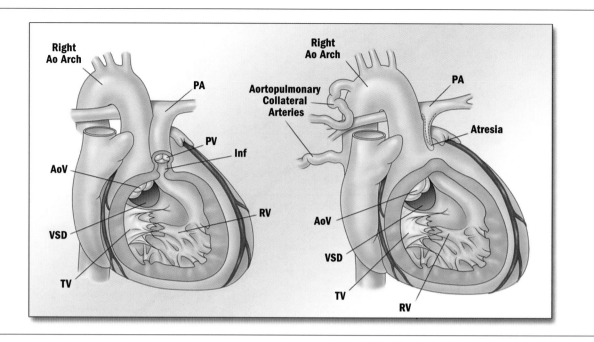

Figure 3

Diagrammatic Representation of Two Variations of Tetralogy of Fallot

The two variations include the more common form with pulmonary stenosis and the more severe form with pulmonary atresia.

Ao = aorta; AoV = aortic valve; Inf = infundibulum; PA = pulmonary artery; PV = pulmonary valve; RV = right ventricle; TV = tricuspid valve; VSD = ventricular septal defect.

Reproduced with permission from Valente AM, Landzberg MJ, Powell AJ. Adult congenital heart disease. In: Libby P, ed. Essential Atlas of Cardiovascular Disease. 4th ed. New York: Current Medicine Group; 2009:241.

Cardiac magnetic resonance (CMR) is an excellent imaging alternative to document the prominent obstructive muscle bundles and relationship to the VSD (*Figure 2*).

Management

Surgical intervention is recommended for any patient with a peak gradient by Doppler >60 mm Hg or a mean gradient >40 mm Hg, regardless of symptoms. Symptomatic patients may be considered for intervention with slighter lower gradients (peak >50 mm Hg, mean >30 mm Hg).[2] Surgical intervention consists of resection of the obstructing muscle bundles, which often includes partial resection of the septal and parietal bands. If a VSD is present, it is closed with a patch or sutures. Additionally, attention must be paid to the left ventricular outflow tract (LVOT), and any subaortic membrane removed at the time of surgery. The long-term outcomes following surgical repair of DCRV are good, with only minimal residual gradients (<10 mm Hg) in the majority of cases.[5]

Key Point

- DCRV is characterized by obstruction at the proximal portion of the os infundibulum, dividing the RV into a high-pressure proximal sinus chamber and a low-pressure distal infundibular chamber.

Tetralogy of Fallot

Definition: Anatomy and Physiology

TOF is a conotruncal anomaly resulting from anterior and leftward deviation of the infundibular septum and is characterized by varying degrees of RVOT obstruction, a VSD, overriding aorta, and RV hypertrophy (*Figure 3*). Children with TOF have varying degrees of cyanosis, based on the amount of RVOT obstruction and right-to-left shunting through the large conoventricular VSD. The majority of adults with TOF will have undergone repair in childhood.

The diagnosis of TOF includes a wide variation in the degrees of RVOT obstruction (*Figure 3*). Patients may have varying degrees of PS or the most severe form of TOF: pulmonary atresia, which occurs in about 15% of cases. Patients with TOF/pulmonary atresia often require several operations to unifocalize the PA segments and to replace the necessary RV-to-PA conduit. Rarely, patients with TOF may have a common AV canal. Rarely, patients with TOF may have an absent pulmonary valve, which is associated with huge branch PAs that may cause bronchial compression.

Types of Surgical Repair

In the late 1950s and 1960s, patients with TOF often underwent palliative procedures, such as a systemic-to-PA

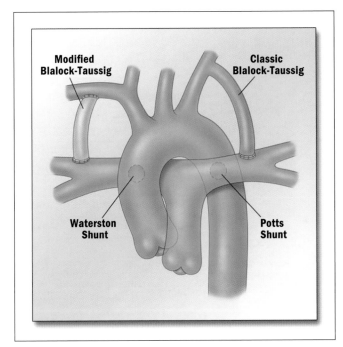

Figure 4a

Diagrammatic Representation of Various Types of Systemic-to-Pulmonary Artery Shunts

Reproduced with permission from Valente AM, Landzberg MJ, Powell AJ. Adult congenital heart disease. In: Libby P, ed. Essential Atlas of Cardiovascular Disease. 4th ed. New York: Current Medicine Group; 2009:242.

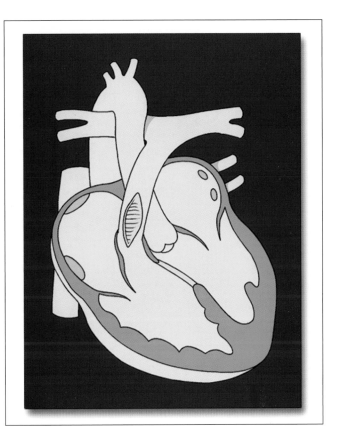

Figure 4b

Diagrammatic Representation of Tetralogy of Fallot Surgical Repair

Modified from Oechslin EN. Echocardiography in Pediatric and Congenital Heart Disease: From Fetus to Adult. Wiley-Blackwell; 2009.

shunt (i.e., the Blalock-Taussig shunt) to augment pulmonary blood flow prior to definitive repair. Various types of palliative shunts are illustrated in *Figure 4a*. Following initial palliation, many patients returned for the definitive repair, which involved surgical relief of RVOT obstruction, most often with a patch of conduit, closure of the VSD, and take-down or closure of the surgical shunt (*Figure 4b*). These procedures often resulted in large right ventriculotomies and destruction of the pulmonary valve, leaving patients with severe PR. Over the past 3 decades, primary repair without initial palliation has been very successful. Surgical strategies now focus on maintaining the integrity of the pulmonary valve and limiting the size of the ventriculotomy. At the time of surgical repair, attention must be paid to the coronary artery anatomy, as 5-10% of patients with TOF have an anomalous left anterior descending (LAD) coronary artery arising from the right sinus of Valsalva or right coronary artery. This anomalous LAD courses across the RVOT and can be inadvertently damaged at the time of repair.

Clinical Exam of the Patient With Repaired Tetralogy of Fallot

The findings on clinical examination of the patient with repaired TOF are reflective of the residual hemodynamic abnormalities. The oxygen saturation is usually normal. A RV heave may be present. The most common murmur is one of PR. This diastolic murmur may not reflect the severity of PR, based on the near equalization of the

diastolic pressures in the RV and PA. It is therefore critically important to note whether the RV volumes are increasing over time when PR is present.

Systolic ejection murmurs of residual RVOT obstruction, including branch PA stenosis, may be present. Signs of right heart failure (elevated jugular venous pressure, lower extremity edema, hepatomegaly) should alert the clinician to failing right heart physiology and warrant further investigation.

Diagnostic Testing of the Patient With Repaired Tetralogy of Fallot

Patients with repaired TOF should have at least an annual follow-up with a cardiologist who has expertise in adult congenital heart disease (ACHD). Annual diagnostic testing should include a 12-lead electrocardiogram. Varying degrees of right bundle branch block are common. A resting QRS duration of >180 msec has been associated with adverse clinical outcomes (sudden death) in this patient population.[6]

In general, asymptomatic adults with repaired TOF should undergo echocardiography at least every 2 years and CMR every 3 years.[7,8] Imaging may be needed more frequently

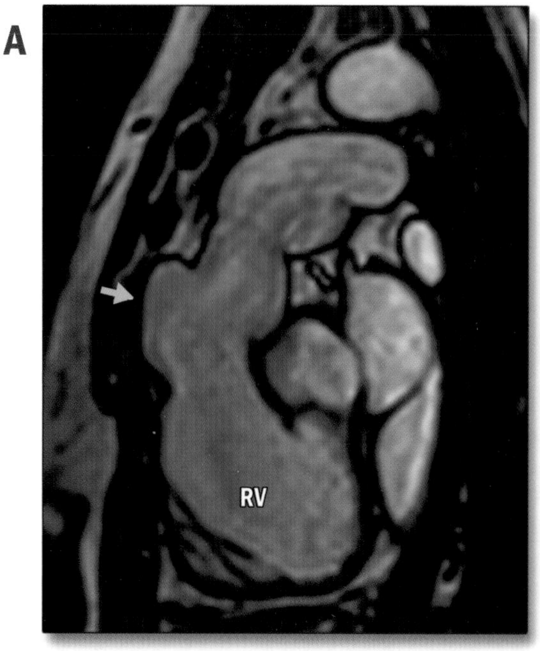

A

RV

Figure 5

Cine Magnetic Resonance Imaging Steady-State Free Precession Image Demonstrating a Right Ventricular Outflow Tract Aneurysm (Arrow) in a Patient With Prior Transannular Patch Repair of Tetralogy of Fallot

RV = right ventricle.

Reproduced with permission from Valente AM, Powell AJ. Clinical applications of cardiovascular magnetic resonance in congenital heart disease. Magn Reson Imaging Clin N Am 2007;15:570.

- Right ventricular dilation and dysfunction.

- Pulmonary regurgitation.

- Tricuspid regurgitation.

- Residual anatomic lesions.
    - Ventricular septal defect.
    - Right ventricular outflow tract obstruction.
    - Branch pulmonary artery stenosis.

- Left ventricular dysfunction (particularly in those with late repair).

- Aortic root dilation (particularly in those with tetralogy of Fallot/pulmonary atresia).

- Arrhythmias (atrial and ventricular).

- Sudden cardiac death.

Table 2

Long-Term Sequelae of Tetralogy of Fallot Surgical Repair

for those patients who are on the verge of fulfilling criteria for pulmonary valve replacement (PVR), have an RV-to-PA conduit, or have demonstrated a substantial worsening of ventricular or clinical parameters on prior studies.[8] CMR is particularly useful in quantifying RV size and function and PR, as well as identifying RVOT aneurysms (*Figure 5*). Periodic cardiopulmonary exercise testing is useful for serial assessment of exercise capacity and to assess for any exercise-induced arrhythmias.

Management of the Patient With Repaired Tetralogy of Fallot

Adults with repaired TOF often have residual hemodynamic problems (*Table 2*). Although pulmonary valve regurgitation is tolerated for many years, the long-term effects of RV volume overload may contribute to ventricular dysfunction and diminished exercise tolerance. Therefore, PVR is a common surgical referral in adults with repaired TOF. Although the indications and optimal timing of PVR in

asymptomatic patients with repaired TOF has not been well established[9] there are Class IIa recommendations for PVR consideration in this population, listed in *Table 3*.[2] Although these recommendations do not include quantitative measurements, great attention has been paid to finding cut-off values by imaging that predict adverse clinical outcomes. Recent data have suggested that patients with repaired TOF should be considered for pulmonary valve replacement prior to a decrease in their ventricular function or an indexed RV end-diastolic volume >150-160 ml/m^2 or an indexed RV end-systolic volume >80 ml/m^2.[10-12]

Patients with repaired TOF have excellent survival into adulthood, with an estimated 0.15% annual risk of sudden cardiac death.[13] Determining predictors of adverse events in these patients is challenging. There may be associated LV dysfunction or a dilated aortic root and aortic regurgitation. The prevalence of atrial and

- Moderate to severe RV dysfunction (Level of Evidence B)

- Moderate to severe RV enlargement (Level of Evidence B)

- Development of symptomatic or sustained atrial or ventricular arrhythmias (Level of Evidence C)

- Moderate to severe tricuspid regurgitation (Level of Evidence C)

Table 3

Class IIa Recommendations for Pulmonary Valve Replacement in Adults With Previous Repair of Tetralogy of Fallot and Severe Pulmonary Regurgitation

RV = right ventricular.

Modified from Warnes CA, Williams RG, Bashore TM, et al. ACC/AHA 2008 guidelines for the management of adults with congenital heart disease: a report of the American College of Cardiology/American Heart Association Task Force on Practice Guidelines (Writing Committee to Develop Guidelines on the Management of Adults With Congenital Heart Disease). Developed in Collaboration With the American Society of Echocardiography, Heart Rhythm Society, International Society for Adult Congenital Heart Disease, Society for Cardiovascular Angiography and Interventions, and Society of Thoracic Surgeons. J Am Coll Cardiol 2008;52:e143-263.

ventricular arrhythmias increases with age.[14] The role of electrophysiology testing in this patient population is not universally established.[15] In a multicenter study of implantable defibrillators in patients with repaired TOF, the only two independent predictors of appropriate shocks were nonsustained ventricular tachycardia on Holter monitoring and a LV end-diastolic pressure of >12 mm Hg.[16]

Key Points

- Common long-term sequelae of TOF repair include PR, RV dilation, and arrhythmias.

- A resting QRS duration of >180 msec is associated with adverse clinical outcomes in patients with repaired TOF.

D-Loop Transposition of the Great Arteries

Definition

D-TGA (D-loop or S,D,D TGA) is a cyanotic heart defect that almost invariably results in death in infancy or early childhood if left untreated. As illustrated in *Figure 6*, this physiology is characterized by ventriculoarterial discordance in which the aorta arises from the RV and the PA arises from the LV. This anatomic arrangement causes blood to circulate in two separate parallel circuits rather than in series. In most cases, the anterior aorta arises from the RV via a subaortic infundibulum, and therefore, there is no continuity between the tricuspid and aortic valves.

Initial survival depends on adequate mixing of the two circulations through an ASD or VSD or patent ductus arteriosus. The most frequently associated anomalies include a VSD (approximately 45%), LVOT obstruction (approximately 25%), and coarctation of the aorta (approximately 5%).

Multiple coronary artery patterns can be seen in patients with TGA. The most commonly occurring coronary artery pattern is one in which the LAD and the left circumflex arises from the left-facing sinus, and the right coronary artery arises from the right-facing sinus. This coronary artery pattern is present in approximately 65% of patients.

Types of Surgical Repair

The initial surgical strategies for TGA were attempted to improve mixing of the parallel circulations at the atrial level. These included the Blalock-Hanlon operation, which involved ASD creation without the use of cardiopulmonary bypass, and the Baffes procedure, which involved inferior vena cava diversion to the left atrium (LA) and right upper pulmonary vein diversion into the right atrium (RA).

Eventually, the balloon atrial septostomy was developed. In this procedure, a catheter is passed across a patent foramen ovale (PFO) into the LA with a balloon. The balloon is inflated, and a larger atrial communication is created as the balloon is pulled back into the RA. This palliation provided improved mixing by creating an ASD until a more definitive repair could be performed.

Many adults with TGA have undergone an atrial switch procedure (*Figure 7a*). Initially pioneered by Mustard in 1959 and Senning in 1964, both of these operations direct the atrial blood flow to the correct ventricles, resulting in restoration of circulations in series. However, this results in the RV as the systemic ventricle, which often becomes dysfunctional later in life. The Mustard procedure involves removal of the atrial septum with reconstruction of the atrial baffles with synthetic material. The Senning operation involves creation of atrial baffles from the patient's intrinsic tissues (i.e., right atrial wall and atrial septum).

The surgical procedure of choice today is the arterial switch operation (ASO) (*Figure 7b*), which results in the LV acting as the systemic ventricle. This involves transection of the aorta and PA above the level of the sinuses. The coronary arteries, including surrounding buttons of aortic wall, are detached from the aorta and sutured into the neoaorta.

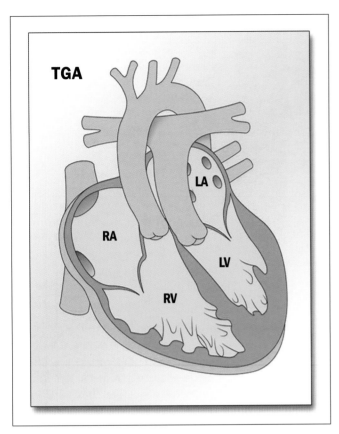

Figure 6

Diagrammatic Representation of the Transposition of the Great Arteries

In this condition, the aorta arises from the right ventricle and the pulmonary artery from the left ventricle. There is AV concordance and ventriculoarterial discordance. Low-oxygen systemic venous blood travels through the right heart, the aorta, the systemic circulation, and then back to the right heart. Oxygenated blood travels through the pulmonary veins, left heart, pulmonary arteries, and then back to the left heart. Thus, the systemic and pulmonary circulations run in parallel rather than in series.

AV = atrioventricular; LA = left atrium; LV = left ventricle; RA = right atrium; RV = right ventricle.

Reproduced with permission from Valente AM, Landzberg MJ, Powell AJ. Adult congenital heart disease. In: Libby P, ed. Essential Atlas of Cardiovascular Disease. 4th ed. New York: Current Medicine Group; 2009:240.

The pulmonary trunk is placed anterior to the aorta and the "switched" great arteries are sutured in place.

Patients with the combination of TGA, VSD, and PS may have undergone a Rastelli procedure (*Figure 7c*). This operation incorporates part of the VSD as the LVOT and directs blood from the VSD to the aorta. It also incorporates part of the VSD as the LVOT and directs blood from the LV to the aorta. This procedure also involves placement of a conduit from the RV to the PA. Although this operation results in restoration of the LV

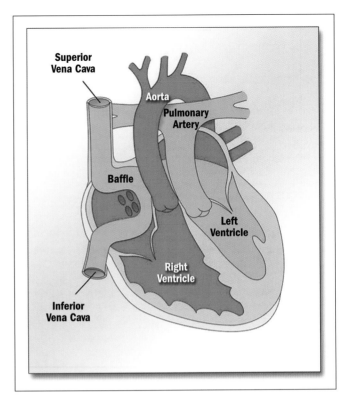

Figure 7a

Atrial Switch Repair (Senning or Mustard Procedure)

With this surgery, systemic and pulmonary venous blood is redirected at the atrial level so that the systemic venous return (low-oxygen blood) flows to the LV and travels out the pulmonary artery, and the pulmonary venous blood (high-oxygen blood) flows to the RV and is ejected out the aorta. As a result, cyanosis is eliminated, but the right ventricle remains in the systemic position.

LV = left ventricle; RV = right ventricle.

Reproduced with permission from Valente AM, Landzberg MJ, Powell AJ. Adult congenital heart disease. In: Libby P, ed. Essential Atlas of Cardiovascular Disease. 4th ed. New York: Current Medicine Group; 2009:240.

as the systemic ventricle, long-term management often involves replacement of the conduit.

Diagnostic Testing of the Postoperative Patient With Transposition of the Great Arteries

The appropriate choice of diagnostic testing of the adult with TGA is dictated by the prior surgical history. *Table 4* lists some of the common sequelae based on prior surgical intervention. In patients with atrial switch procedures, echocardiographic evaluation for residual atrial-level shunts can be accomplished with a contrast injection with agitated saline. Transesphogeal echocardiography is also helpful in defining atrial baffle leaks or obstructions. Evaluation of systemic RV dysfunction can be particularly challenging by echocardiography because of limited acoustic windows and the complex geometry of the RV. CMR

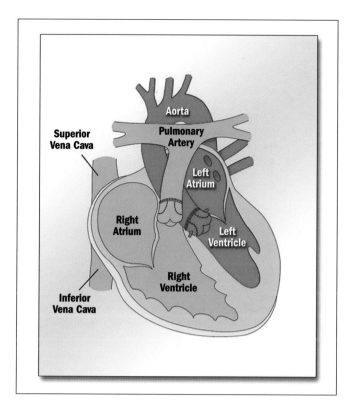

Figure 7b
Arterial Switch Operation

In this procedure, the ascending aorta and main pulmonary arteries are transected and then attached to the concordant ventricle, and the coronary arteries are detached and transferred to the new aortic root. In order to minimize kinking of the pulmonary arteries, the right pulmonary artery is often positioned anterior to the ascending aorta (LeCompte maneuver). This surgery both eliminates cyanosis and establishes the left ventricle as the systemic ventricle.

Reproduced with permission from Valente AM, Landzberg MJ, Powell AJ. Adult congenital heart disease. In: Libby P, ed. Essential Atlas of Cardiovascular Disease. 4th ed. New York: Current Medicine Group; 2009:241.

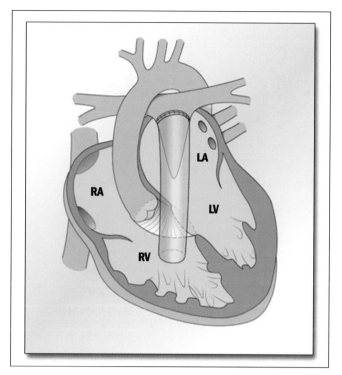

Figure 7c
Rastelli procedure

Patients with TGA, a ventricular septal defect, and significant pulmonary stenosis often undergo a Rastelli operation because an arterial switch operation would leave them with an obstructed left ventricular outflow tract. A Rastelli operation involves patch closure of the ventricular septal defect to baffle left ventricular blood to the aorta, placement of a right ventricular to pulmonary artery conduit, and oversewing of the proximal main pulmonary artery.

LA = left atrium; LV = left ventricle; RA = right atrium; RV = right ventricle.

Reproduced with permission from Valente AM, Landzberg MJ, Powell AJ. Adult congenital heart disease. In: Libby P, ed. Essential Atlas of Cardiovascular Disease. 4th ed. New York: Current Medicine Group; 2009:241.

and computed tomography are increasingly being used in the diagnostic evaluation of these patients to provide quantitative assessment of systemic RV size and function. These advanced imaging modalities are also useful in patients status/post ASO who may have proximal branch PA stenosis or neoaortic root dilation. The diagnostic testing for patients status/ post ASO also must include assessment for coronary artery patency. Often, this can be accomplished noninvasively; however, invasive coronary angiography is reasonable in adults with TGA/ASO to rule out coronary artery obstruction. This is a Class IIa recommendation in the ACC/AHA 2008 Guidelines for Management of Adults with Congenital Heart Disease.[2]

Management
Annual follow-up with a cardiologist experienced in the management of ACHD is recommended. Atrial arrhythmias are common in adults who have undergone the atrial switch procedure and are associated with increased risk of sudden cardiac death in this population.[17] Patients with Mustard or Senning procedures have a high incidence of sinus node dysfunction, and those with sinus bradycardia should be considered for permanent pacemaker placement. Consultation with an electrophysiologist experienced in the care of adults with CHD is warranted.

One of the largest concerns in patients who have previously undergone atrial switch procedures is progressive systemic RV dysfunction. However, the reported prevalence varies widely in the literature. The medical management of systemic RV dysfunction has not

Arterial Switch	Rastelli Operation	Atrial Switch
Arterial anastomosis stenosis	RV-PA conduit obstruction	Systemic venous baffle obstruction
Branch PA stenosis	Pulmonary regurgitation	Pulmonary venous baffle obstruction
Coronary artery stenosis	Subaortic stenosis	Baffle leak
LV dysfunction	Ventricular dysfunction	Systemic RV dysfunction
Aortic root dilation		Tricuspid regurgitation
Aortic regurgitation		LVOT obstruction

Table 4

Potential Long-Term Sequelae Following Various Surgical Palliations for Complete Transposition of the Great Arteries

LV = left ventricular;
LVOT = left ventricular outflow tract;
PA = pulmonary artery;
RV = right ventricular.

been well validated. In one multicenter study, the use of angiotensin-receptor blockade was not associated with improved exercise capacity in these patients.

Interventional catheterization often plays an important role in adults with TGA. Specifically, in atrial switch patients, it may be beneficial to occlude residual baffle leaks or dilate/stent stenotic systemic or pulmonary atrial baffles. In TGA patients status/post ASO, catheterization may be used to dilate or stent supravalvular or branch PA stenosis. In patients with a Rastelli repair, dilation and/or stent placement in RV to PA conduits and device closure of residual VSD can be accomplished. The AHA/ACC 2008 guidelines list Class I indications for repeat surgical interventions in patients with TGA.[2]

Key Point

- Long-term complications of the atrial switch procedure for TGA include systemic RV dysfunction, TR, systemic and pulmonary venous baffle obstruction, baffle leaks, and atrial arrhythmias.

L-Loop Transposition of the Great Arteries ("Physiologically Corrected" Transposition of the Great Arteries)

Definition

Physiologically corrected TGA (L-loop or S,L,L TGA, also referred to as congenitally corrected TGA) is an uncommon congenital heart lesion and is characterized by both AV and ventriculoarterial discordance (*Figure 8*). In this physiology, the systemic venous return is directed into the RA, which is connected by a mitral valve into the LV. The LA receives the pulmonary venous blood from the pulmonary veins and is connected to the RV by a tricuspid valve. The aorta arises from the morphological RV and the PA from the LV. This results in normal systemic arterial oxygenation; however, the RV is the systemic ventricle in this arrangement. This diagnosis may be made for the first time in adulthood, particularly in patients without associated lesions.

Associated Lesions

Dextrocardia may be present in up to 20% of patients with physiologically corrected TGA. Associated lesions are common and include VSD (approximately 70%), tricuspid valve abnormalities (approximately 50%), and PS (approximately 30%). Malformations of the morphological tricuspid valve (i.e., systemic AV valve) are common, including Ebstein anomaly. However, the valve appearance is distinctly different from classic Ebstein anomaly, as in patients with physiologically corrected TGA, the tricuspid valve does not exhibit the large, sail-like anterior leaflet and little, if any, atrialized portion of the RV.

The usual coronary artery pattern is described as "inverted." The right coronary artery has the epicardial distribution of a normal left coronary artery, bifurcating into an anterior descending and circumflex artery, which runs posteriorly in the right AV groove. The left-sided coronary artery courses into the left AV groove.

Coronary venous anatomy is also variable. The coronary sinus develops from the left horn of the sinus venous resulting in drainage to the morphological RA. However, the venous branches, including the great cardiac vein, develop with the morphological ventricles, which are inverted. Understanding these differences and documenting these findings with imaging is particularly important prior to electrophysiological interventions involving device placement. There are abnormalities in the conduction system, and the incidence of complete heart block in adulthood is up to 2% per year.

Management

Many adults with physiologically corrected TGA consider themselves to be asymptomatic. However, up to two-thirds of patients with associated cardiac lesions and one-quarter of those without associated lesions have congestive heart failure. Congestive heart failure is defined by physical exam findings of pulmonary edema, hepatomegaly, or a ventricular gallop. It also can be identified from the need for diuretics or afterload reduction medications. Despite their perceived asymptomatic status, objective exercise testing reveals that peak workload is greatly diminished in these patients (i.e., 38% of normal values).

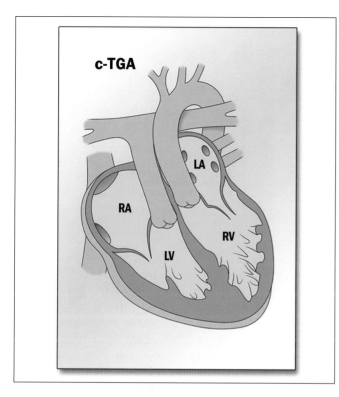

Figure 8

Diagrammatic Representation of the Most Common Form of Physiologically Corrected Transposition of the Great Arteries

c-TGA is characterized by both atrioventricular and ventriculoarterial discordance. Systemic venous blood passes from the right atrium through the mitral valve into the morphologic left ventricle to the pulmonary artery. Oxygenated blood then returns from the lungs to the left atrium through the tricuspid valve into the morphologic right ventricle and then out the aorta.

c-TGA = corrected transposition of the great arteries; LA = left atrium; LV = left ventricle; RA = right atrium; RV = right ventricle.

Reproduced with permission from Valente AM, Landzberg MJ, Powell AJ. Adult congenital heart disease. In: Libby P, ed. Essential Atlas of Cardiovascular Disease. 4th ed. New York: Current Medicine Group; 2009:239.

In one multicenter study of 182 patients with physiologically corrected TGA, systemic RV dysfunction was common and was moderate or severe in more than 30% of cases. Multiple mechanisms for systemic RV dysfunction have been proposed, including coronary perfusion mismatch. Fixed myocardial perfusion defects at rest and with exercise have been demonstrated, and the extent of perfusion defects correlates inversely with the ejection fraction.

Medical management for the failing systemic RV in patients with physiologically corrected TGA has not been well established. There are recent reports that cardiac resynchronization therapy has led to some improvement in functional class, peak oxygen consumption, and ventricular function. However, long-term data are lacking.

Tricuspid regurgitation ([TR] or systemic AV valve regurgitation) is common in adults with physiologically corrected TGA and may be the consequence of a combination of mechanisms, including tricuspid annular dilation, leaflet malcoaptation, or RV dilation. In one study of 40 patients with physiologically corrected TGA, those with significant TR were 14.8-times more likely to die than those without significant TR. The median time from onset of TR to RV failure was 5 years. Therefore, many centers advocate for replacement of the tricuspid valve at the earliest signs of ventricular dysfunction. A recent retrospective analysis from the Mayo Clinic identified preoperative RV ejection fraction to be the only independent predictor of postoperative ejection fraction 1 year following tricuspid valve replacement.[18]

Some adults with physiologically corrected TGA will have undergone a "physiologic repair" earlier in life with the goal of addressing any of the associated defects, while leaving the RV as the systemic ventricle. However, this approach is associated with significant morbidity and mortality. Newer surgical approaches have been developed to create an "anatomical repair" with the goal of addressing any associated defects and allowing the LV to be the systemic ventricle. These approaches include: a double switch operation, an atrial switch and Rastelli operation, or a hemi-Mustard/bidirectional Glenn and an arterial switch.

Current management guidelines for adults with physiologically corrected TGA call for regular follow-up. This should include echocardiography-Doppler and/or CMR performed yearly or at least every other year by staff trained in imaging complex CHD. If progression of heart block is suspected, ambulatory electrocardiogram monitoring for 24 hours should be considered.[2]

Key Point

- Patients with physiologically corrected TGA may not be diagnosed until adulthood. These patients may present with complete heart block, systemic RV dysfunction, or TR.

Double Outlet Right Ventricle

Definition: Anatomy and Physiology

DORV is a unique type of conotruncal anomaly in which both great arteries are completely or nearly completely aligned with the RV. This is a complex form of CHD and has controversial nomenclature regarding the best classification system. Some centers advocate the "50% rule," which occurs when more than 50% of the semilunar valve is related to that ventricle over a VSD. This designation may be somewhat arbitrary and imprecise. DORV encompasses a variety of anatomical and physiological arrangements, ranging from physiology that resembles a VSD to TOF to TGA.

There is great heterogeneity in the clinical presentation of patients with DORV. The location of the VSD is almost always in the same location—in the "Y" of the septal band. The VSD size, relationship of the VSD to the great arteries, conal morphology, presence of outflow tract (OT) obstruction, and associated cardiovascular defects primarily determine the physiology. The VSD may be subaortic (approximately 50%), subpulmonary (approximately 30%), doubly committed (approximately 10%), or noncommitted or remote (approximately 20%). In DORV, there are various possibilities for conal morphology, including bilateral conus, subpulmonary conus, subaortic conus, and bilaterally absent conus. The great arteries relationships are also variable, depending on the semilunar valves relation to each other. Potential great artery relationships include: side-by-side, normally related, D-malposition, L-malposition, and a directly anterior aortic valve or posterior and leftward aortic valve. There are four common physiological variations of DORV (*Figure 9*, panels A, B, C, D) that dictate the clinical presentation and approach to surgical repair. These include:

1. VSD physiology: DORV with large VSD and no PS

2. TOF physiology: DORV with subaortic VSD and PS

3. TGA physiology: DORV with subpulmonary VSD ± aortic obstruction

4. Single-ventricle physiology: DORV with mitral atresia or significant ventricular hypoplasia

A specific subset of DORV patients with subpulmonary VSD, bilateral conus, and side-by-side semilunar valves is known as "Taussig-Bing" anomaly. These patients often require frequent interventions in adult life to address residual obstruction in both OTs.[19]

Associated Lesions
OT obstruction occurs in up to 70% of DORV patients; the most common form is pulmonary OT obstruction in the presence of a subaortic VSD. Subaortic stenosis or aortic arch obstruction occurs in up to 50% of cases with a subpulmonary VSD.

DORV patients also may have abnormalities of the AV valves, including a common AV valve (AV canal defect).

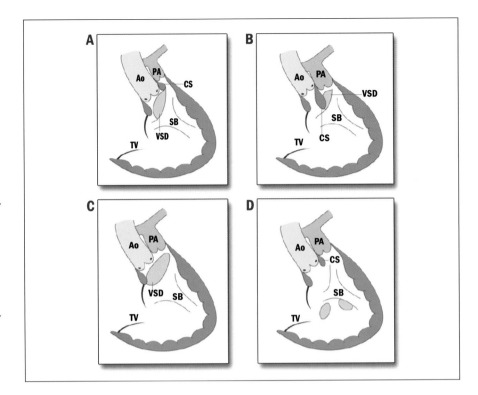

Figure 9

Diagrammatic Representation of the Most Common Forms of Double Outlet Right Ventricle

Panel A: Subaortic VSD. **Panel B**: Subpulmonic VSD. **Panel C**: Doubly committed VSD. **Panel D**: Remote VSD.

Ao = aorta; CS = coronary sinus; PA = pulmonary artery; SB = side branch; TV = tricuspid valve; VSD = ventricular septal defect.

Reproduced with permission from Lopez L. Double outlet ventricles. In: Lai WW, Mertens LL, Cohen MS, Geva T, eds. Echocardiography in Pediatric and Congenital Heart Disease: From Fetus to Adult. Wiley-Blackwell; 2009.

Abnormalities of the mitral valve are associated with worse outcomes, as a straddling mitral valve may complicate surgical repair. DORV with mitral valve atresia requires surgical management down a single-ventricle pathway.

DORV also may be associated with ASDs, persistent left superior vena cava, and left juxtaposition of the atrial appendages. DORV is common in patients with asplenia-type of heterotaxy syndrome.

Management
The surgical approach to DORV depends on the intracardiac anatomy. The position of the VSD and relationship to the great arteries is critical to the surgical approach. In the most common form (subaortic VSD), the surgical goals include establishing LV to aortic continuity by patching the VSD to tunnel the LV to the aorta. This pathway is often long and tortuous and in some cases, the VSD must be enlarged to create this tunnel. Care must be taken to avoid creation of LVOT obstruction, which may result in the need for reoperation. If there is PS, relief of obstruction must be accomplished by either patch

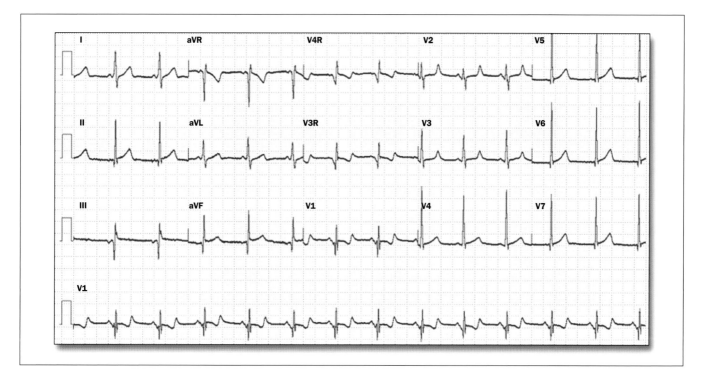

Figure 10

Twelve-Lead Electrocardiogram in a Patient With Ebstein Anomaly

Note the subtle pre-excitation and the relatively narrow QRS because the right-sided pathway tends to pseudonormalize the intrinsic RBBB present in most of these patients.

RBBB = right bundle branch block.

Image courtesy of Douglas Mah, MD, Boston Children's Hospital, Department of Cardiology, Boston, MA.

---

enlargement of the RVOT, valvotomy, or insertion of a conduit to establish RV to PA continuity.

For patients with DORV and a subpulmonary VSD, the surgical repair is similar to those with D-loop TGA with a baffle from the LV to the pulmonary valve and ASO. For patients with unfavorable anatomy for a biventricular repair, patients are staged to a Fontan palliation.

> **Key Point**
>
> - In patients with DORV, the VSD size, relationship of the VSD to the great arteries, conal morphology, presence of OT obstruction, and associated cardiovascular defects primarily determine the physiology.

Ebstein Anomaly

Definition: Anatomy and Physiology
Ebstein anomaly is a rare congenital heart defect that includes a wide spectrum of anatomical and functional abnormalities of the RV and tricuspid valve.[20] Genetic factors contributing to Ebstein anomaly is not well understood; however, mutations in the transcription factor NKX2.5, 10p13-14 deletion, and 1p34.3-36.11 deletion have been described. The morphologic defect of Ebstein anomaly involves failure of delamination of the tricuspid valve leaflets, causing adherence of the leaflets to the RV myocardium. This results in apical and posterior displacement of the dilated tricuspid valve annulus. The anterior leaflet is often redundant and thickened, and is often referred to as "sail-like" in appearance. Chordal attachments may result in tethering of the valve, which results in restricted leaflet motion. The displacement of the functional valve annulus results in an "atrialized" portion of the RV, which has tissue properties of an RV but is physiologically part of the atrium. The abnormal tricuspid valve is often regurgitant and rarely stenotic.[21]

The clinical presentation of Ebstein anomaly is highly variable, both in the age at presentation and clinical course, and depends on the anatomic and physiological severity of the disease. Neonates with a poorly functioning RV and severely dysfunctional tricuspid valve may present with heart failure and/or cyanosis. Children with milder forms of valvular pathology and good RV function may not present until later in life. The clinical presentation in adults can range from an asymptomatic state to severe right heart failure or arrhythmias. Symptoms depend on several factors, including the extent of tricuspid valve leaflet

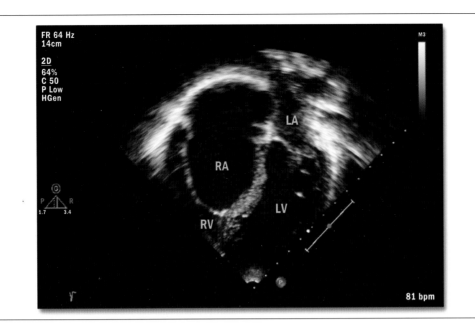

Figure 11

Apical Four-Chamber Echocardiographic View of a Patient With Ebstein Anomaly

The tricuspid valve is apically displaced from the tricuspid valve annular plane.

LA = left atrium; LV = left ventricle; RA = right atrium; RV = right ventricle.

distortion, degree of TR, right atrial pressure, and presence of a right-to-left atrial shunt.

Clinical Exam and Associated Lesions

The clinical examination findings may include an RV lift, loud first heart sound with systolic clicks, and a holosystolic murmur of TR. The crisp, snapping sound that quickly follows the first heart sound is referred to as a "sail sign," exemplifying the snap of the redundant anterior leaflet of the tricuspid valve. It is so-called as it is likened to the unfurling of a sail on a sailboat. The jugular venous pressure is often normal, despite significant TR as a result of the large compliant RA. Cyanosis may be present if there is an associated atrial-level shunt, which is common in this condition. Specifically, ASD and PFO predispose patients to paradoxical emboli and right-to-left shunting. Patients with Ebstein anomaly and atrial-level shunts may not be cyanotic at rest, but become cyanotic with exertion.

Patients may have additional anatomical lesions such as PS, mitral valve prolapse, coarctation of the aorta, or LV noncompaction.

As noted earlier, Ebstein-like valve abnormalities commonly are seen in the systemic ventricle of patients with physiologically corrected TGA.

Atrial arrhythmias are common, with concealed accessory pathways present in approximately 50% of these patients, and Wolff-Parkinson White (WPW) syndrome is present in at least 20% of Ebstein patients. The majority of accessory pathways are right-sided and located in the right posterior and posteroseptal regions (*Figure 10*). In patients with L-loop transposition, the pre-excitation will accompany the systemic ventricle. Multiple accessory pathways may be present in individual patients.

Diagnostic Testing

Chest radiograph demonstrates an enlarged cardiothoracic ratio. TTE is essential in assessing the valve morphology and degree of TR. Echocardiographic criteria for Ebstein anomaly includes that the septal leaflet insertion site is apically displaced >0.8 cm/m^2 relative to the anterior mitral valve leaflet insertion site (*Figure 11*). The septal and posterior leaflets may be thickened, dysplastic, and muscularized. In severe forms, the posterior leaflet may be displaced. The anterior leaflet is elongated, redundant, and often fenestrated with restricted leaflet motion. Most adults with Ebstein anomaly have at least moderate TR. Severe RA and RV dilation are common. Three-dimensional echocardiography displays the "en face" view of the tricuspid valve and demonstrates tethering of the leaflets to the RV free wall. The assessment of RV systolic performance may be challenging with TTE because of the complex, nongeometric shape of the RV. CMR can provide quantitative analysis of the ventricular size and function as well as determine the amount of TR and degree of intracardiac shunting.[22] Objective cardiopulmonary exercise testing may be useful to document any cyanosis as a result of a right-to-left shunt and exercise capacity.[23]

Management

Patients with Ebstein anomaly should undergo periodic evaluations by cardiologists with expertise in ACHD (*Table 5*). The late survival of unoperated adults with Ebstein anomaly is reported at 76% at 10 years and 41% at 20 years. Multivariate predictors of cardiac-related death include male gender, cardiothoracic ratio ≥0.65, and the severity of TV leaflet displacement.

Medical therapies in Ebstein anomaly patients are largely directed at alleviating heart failure symptoms and controlling arrhythmias. At this time, there is no evidence that medical therapies for Ebstein anomaly improve

Particular attention should be paid to the following:

- Cyanotic patients
- Substantial cardiomegaly (cardiothoracic ratio >64%)
- RV function, which may worsen and cause congestion
- TR or tricuspid stenosis in a previously operated patient
- Degeneration and/or infection of a bioprosthetic valve, or thrombosis and/or infection of a mechanical valve
- Recurrent atrial arrhythmias
- Ventricular arrhythmias
- Complete heart block

Table 5

Periodic Evaluation for Patients With Ebstein Anomaly

RV = right ventricular; TR = tricuspid regurgitation.

Modified from Silversides CK, Kiess M, Beauchesne L, et al. Canadian Cardiovascular Society 2009 Consensus Conference on the management of adults with congenital heart disease: outflow tract obstruction, coarctation of the aorta, tetralogy of Fallot, Ebstein anomaly, and Marfan's syndrome. Can J Cardiol 2010;26:e80-97, and Warnes CA, Williams RG, Bashore TM, et al. ACC/AHA 2008 guidelines for the management of adults with congenital heart disease: a report of the American College of Cardiology/American Heart Association Task Force on Practice Guidelines (Writing Committee to Develop Guidelines on the Management of Adults With Congenital Heart Disease). Developed in Collaboration With the American Society of Echocardiography, Heart Rhythm Society, International Society for Adult Congenital Heart Disease, Society for Cardiovascular Angiography and Interventions, and Society of Thoracic Surgeons. J Am Coll Cardiol 2008;52:e143-263.

mortality; therefore, therapies are reserved largely for symptomatic patients.

Percutaneous closure of ASD/PFO to relieve right-to-left shunting may be beneficial in select cases of patients with Ebstein anomaly with preserved RV function and minimal TR.[24]

Patients with symptomatic arrhythmias should undergo electrophysiological study, and if indicated, radiofrequency ablation. There is a lower rate of success for catheter ablation and a greater risk of recurrent arrhythmias in Ebstein anomaly patients compared with those patients with structurally normal hearts.

Surgical options for Ebstein anomaly are directed at restoring tricuspid valve competence, reducing right heart size, and closing atrial-level shunts.[25] The surgical techniques for tricuspid valve repair have evolved over time and repair is preferable to tricuspid valve replacement. Several anatomical features are associated with a favorable repair and include a large, mobile anterior leaflet with a free leading edge, presence of adequate septal leaflet tissue, and delamination of the inferior leaflet. Whereas tethering of the

leaflet makes the repair more difficult. When tricuspid valve repair is not possible, bioprosthetic valve replacement is a reasonable option for adults with Ebstein anomaly.

In select patients with severe RV dysfunction or cases with tricuspid valve stenosis (mean gradient >6 mm Hg), a bidirectional cavopulmonary shunt (Glenn shunt) may be preformed, providing the pulmonary vascular resistance is low. This "one-and-a-half ventricle" procedure can reduce the volume of the RV by as much as 35-45%. However, patients may experience some side effects including pulsatile head and neck veins, facial swelling, and development of arteriovenous malformations.

Key Points

- Ebstein anomaly is a rare congenital heart defect and the age at presentation is related to the severity of the disease, with more severe disease presenting earlier in life. Up to 20% have evidence for WPW syndrome. An examination, electrocardiogram, and chest X-ray may provide clues to the diagnosis. The echocardiogram is more definitive, and requires the apical displacement of the septal leaflet >20 mm (>8 mm/m^2) and the presence of a redundant elongated anterior TV leaflet.

- A PFO or ASD is common in >50% of patients with Ebstein anomaly and leads to exercise hypoxemia.

- The indications for surgical intervention in Ebstein anomaly include symptoms or deteriorating exercise capacity.

References

1. Lin AE, Basson CT, Goldmuntz E, et al. Adults with genetic syndromes and cardiovascular abnormalities: clinical history and management. Genet Med 2008;10:469-94.

2. Warnes CA, Williams RG, Bashore TM, et al. ACC/AHA 2008 Guidelines for the Management of Adults With Congenital Heart Disease: a report of the American College of Cardiology/American Heart Association Task Force on Practice Guidelines (Writing Committee to Develop Guidelines on the Management of Adults With Congenital Heart Disease). Developed in Collaboration With the American Society of Echocardiography, Heart Rhythm Society, International Society for Adult Congenital Heart Disease, Society for Cardiovascular Angiography and Interventions, and Society of Thoracic Surgeons. J Am Coll Cardiol 2008;52:e143-263.

3. Qian X, Qian Y, Zhou Y, Yang X. Percutaneous pulmonary balloon valvuloplasty provides good long-term outcomes in adults with pulmonary valve stenosis. J Invasive Cardiol 2015;27:E291-6.

4. Oliver JM, Garrido A, Gonzalez A, et al. Rapid progression of midventricular obstruction in adults with double-chambered right ventricle. J Thorac Cardiovasc Surg 2003;126:711-7.

5. Hachiro Y, Takagi N, Koyanagi T, Morikawa M, Abe T. Repair of double-chambered right ventricle: surgical results and long-term follow-up. Ann Thorac Surg 2001;72:1520-2.

6. Gatzoulis MA, Balaji S, Webber SA, et al. Risk factors for arrhythmia and sudden cardiac death late after repair of tetralogy of Fallot: a multicentre study. Lancet 2000;356:975-81.

7. Valente AM, Cook S, Festa P, et al. Multimodality imaging guidelines for patients with repaired tetralogy of Fallot: a report from the American Society of Echocardiography: developed in collaboration with the Society for Cardiovascular Magnetic Resonance and the Society for Pediatric Radiology. J Am Soc Echocardiogr 2014;27:111-41.

8. Wald RM, Valente AM, Gauvreau K, et al. Cardiac magnetic resonance markers of progressive RV dilation and dysfunction after tetralogy of Fallot repair. Heart 2015;101:1724-30.

9. Geva T. Repaired tetralogy of Fallot: the roles of cardiovascular magnetic resonance in evaluating pathophysiology and for pulmonary valve replacement decision support. J Cardiovasc Magn Reson 2011;13:9.

10. Lee C, Lee CH, Kwak JG, et al. Factors associated with right ventricular dilatation and dysfunction in patients with chronic pulmonary regurgitation after repair of tetralogy of Fallot: analysis of magnetic resonance imaging data from 218 patients. J Thorac Cardiovasc Surg 2014;148:2589-95.

11. Bokma JP, Winter MM, Oosterhof T, et al. Preoperative thresholds for mid-to-late haemodynamic and clinical outcomes after pulmonary valve replacement in tetralogy of Fallot. Eur Heart J 2016;37;829-35.

12. Geva T. Indications for pulmonary valve replacement in repaired tetralogy of Fallot: the quest continues. Circulation 2013;128:1855-7.

13. Khairy P, Dore A, Poirier N, et al. Risk stratification in surgically repaired tetralogy of Fallot. Expert Rev Cardiovasc Ther 2009;7:755-62.

14. Khairy P, Aboulhosn J, Gurvitz MZ, et al. Arrhythmia burden in adults with surgically repaired tetralogy of Fallot: a multi-institutional study. Circulation 2010;122:868-75.

15. Khairy P, Landzberg MJ, Gatzoulis MA, et al. Value of programmed ventricular stimulation after tetralogy of Fallot repair: a multicenter study. Circulation 2004;109:1994-2000.

16. Khairy P, Harris L, Landzberg MJ, et al. Implantable cardioverter-defibrillators in tetralogy of Fallot. Circulation 2008;117:363-70.

17. Kammeraad JA, van Deurzen CH, Sreeram N, et al. Predictors of sudden cardiac death after Mustard or Senning repair for transposition of the great arteries. J Am Coll Cardiol 2004;44:1095-102.

18. Mongeon FP, Connolly HM, Dearani JA, Li Z, Warnes CA. Congenitally corrected transposition of the great arteries ventricular function at the time of systemic atrioventricular valve replacement predicts long-term ventricular function. J Am Coll Cardiol 2011;57:2008-17.

19. Schwarz F, Blaschczok HC, Sinzobahamvya N, et al. The Taussig-Bing anomaly: long-term results. Eur J Cardiothorac Surg 2013;44:821-7.

20. Dearani JA, Mora BN, Nelson TJ, Haile DT, O'Leary PW. Ebstein anomaly review: what's now, what's next? Expert Rev Cardiovasc Ther 2015;13:1101-9.

21. Frescura C, Angelini A, Daliento L, Thiene G. Morphological aspects of Ebstein's anomaly in adults. Thorac Cardiovasc Surg 2000;48:203-8.

22. Yalonetsky S, Tobler D, Greutmann M, et al. Cardiac magnetic resonance imaging and the assessment of Ebstein anomaly in adults. Am J Cardiol 2011;107:767-73.

23. Tobler D, Yalonetsky S, Crean AM, et al. Right heart characteristics and exercise parameters in adults with Ebstein anomaly: new perspectives from cardiac magnetic resonance imaging studies. Int J Cardiol 2013;165:146-50.

24. Silva M, Teixeira A, Menezes I, et al. Percutaneous closure of atrial right-to-left shunt in patients with Ebstein's anomaly of the tricuspid valve. EuroIntervention 2012;8:94-7.

25. Attenhofer Jost CH, Connolly HM, Scott CG, Burkhart HM, Warnes CA, Dearani JA. Outcome of cardiac surgery in patients 50 years of age or older with ebstein anomaly: survival and functional improvement. J Am Coll Cardiol 2012;59:2101-6.

Congenital Heart Disease

Coronary Artery Anomalies and Fistulas

Background and Incidence

Coronary anomalies are a rare entity. In an analysis of one cardiac catheterization database including 126,595 patients, there were 1,886 reported coronary anomalies, which was 1.3% of the patients in this large cohort.[1]

Several classification schemes have been developed over the years. One of the early schemes suggested classification into minor, major, and secondary anomalies based on differences from the normal vessel space.[2] Additional systems of classification based on embryology and how the coronary anomaly differs from the normal vessel have been published.[3,4] In this review, we will focus on the clinical implications of coronary anomalies and discuss anomalies which are considered benign and those considered to have potentially serious clinical complications.

In the normal configuration, coronary anatomy is comprised of three main arteries (*Figure 1*). The left anterior descending (LAD) courses in the anterior interventricular groove on the epicardial surface of the heart between the left and right ventricles. The LAD gives off smaller branches designated as septal perforators, which perfuse the ventricular septum, and diagonal branches, which supply the myocardium of the anterolateral wall of the left ventricular. The size of these branches varies in normal anatomy. The left circumflex artery (LCX) courses in the AV groove on the epicardial surface of the heart between the left atrium and left ventricle.

Todd L. Kiefer, MD, FACC
This author has nothing to disclose.

Learner Objectives

Upon completion of this module, the reader will be able to:
1. Define the classification of coronary anomalies.
2. Recognize coronary anomalies associated with congenital heart disease.
3. Summarize which coronary anomalies are considered benign and those which have potential for adverse clinical events.
4. Describe the guideline recommendations for management of coronary anomalies.

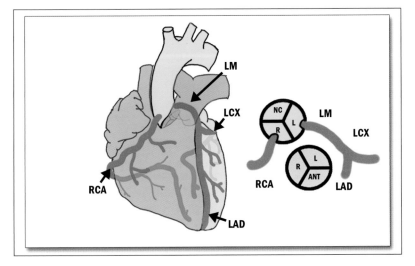

Figure 1
Normal Coronary Anatomy

ANT = anterior; L = left; LAD = left anterior descending; LCX = left circumflex; LM = left main; NC = noncoronary sinus of Valsalva; R = right; RCA = right coronary artery.

Image courtesy of Thomas Bashore, MD, ACCSAP 8.

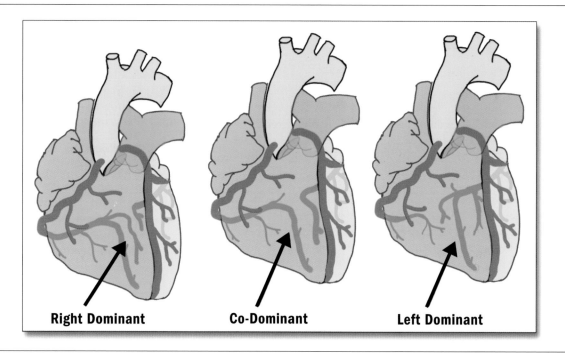

Figure 2
Coronary Dominance Definitions

Image courtesy of Thomas Bashore, MD, ACCSAP 8.

One or more obtuse marginal branches may be present perfusing the lateral wall myocardium. In addition, some individuals have a branch as part of the normal anatomic spectrum designated as a ramus intermedius branch, originating at the distal aspect of the left main between the LAD and LCX. Finally, the right coronary artery (RCA) courses in the AV groove on the epicardial surface of the heart between the right atrium and right ventricle. Branches from the RCA include a conus branch, a right ventricular branch, and an acute marginal branch. If the RCA also gives off a posterior descending artery (PDA) branch perfusing the posterior aspect of the interventricular septum and posterolateral (PL) branches perfusing the posterior myocardium of the left ventricle, then right dominant coronary circulation is present (*Figure 2*). This is the most common configuration, present in 90% of the population.[3]

Codominant coronary circulation is present when the RCA gives rise to a PDA branch and no PL branches. This anatomy is present in approximately 2.5% of the population.[3] When the PDA originates after the PL branches from the most distal aspect of the LCX, then left dominant coronary circulation is present. Occasionally, other variations are present, such as a large LAD wrapping around the apex of the heart to serve the PDA myocardial territory or a large acute marginal branch from the RCA extending to the PDA territory. Additional coronary branches include the sinus nodal artery and AV nodal artery. The artery to the sinus node arises from the RCA in approximately 55% of the population and from the LCX

in 45%. The AV nodal artery originates from the RCA or LCX depending on which vessel gives rise to the PDA.

An important concept to understand and characterize coronary anomalies is the origin of the coronary arteries from the sinuses of Valsalva. In normal anatomy, a left main stem arises from the left sinus of Valsalva and bifurcates into the LAD and LCX branches as previously detailed. Likewise, the RCA arises from the right sinus of Valsalva. This will be explored further with discussion of the important concept of anomalous coronary arteries from the opposite sinus of Valsalva.

Coronary blood flow is determined by the difference between the aortic diastolic pressure and the ventricular end-diastolic pressure. This is often referred to as the coronary perfusion pressure. For the left coronary artery system, most flow is during diastole. However, because right ventricular systolic pressure is low under normal physiologic conditions, the RCA is perfused during both systole and diastole.

Key Point

- Coronary artery anomalies are rare, being observed in approximately 1% of catheterizations.

- **Anomalies of Coronary Origin**
  - **No other congenital heart disease**
    - Separate orifice for conus artery
    - Separate LAD and LCX ostia
    - Circumflex artery from the RCA or right sinus of Valsalva
    - Abnormal origin of RCA or LM within their respective cusps (high or low origin)
    - Anomalous RCA, LM, or LAD with a course anterior to the pulmonary artery
  - **Other congenital heart disease**
    - Tetralogy of Fallot: origin of LAD from RCA or right sinus of Valsalva
    - D-transposition of great arteries: origin of RCA or both RCA and LCX from posterior cusp
- **Anomalies of Coronary Course**
  - Myocardial bridging (intramyocardial vessel course) without documented ischemia
- **Anomalies of the Vessel Wall**
  - Coronary ectasia
  - Small or moderate-sized coronary artery aneurysm
- **Anomalies of Coronary Destination**
  - Small coronary fistula
  - Thebesian veins draining to the left ventricle

Table 1

Common Coronary Artery Anomalies That Rarely Result in Clinical Consequences

LAD = left anterior descending; LCX = left circumflex; LM = left main; RCA = right coronary artery.

Benign Coronary Anomalies

Table 1 describes coronary artery anomalies that usually are without clinical consequence.

Coronary Artery Origin Anomalies

The most common anomaly of coronary origin is the conus artery originating from a distinct ostium in the right sinus of Valsalva and not from the RCA, which is observed in approximately 50% of the population. Next, less commonly, instead of a left main trunk giving rise to the LAD and LCX, there are distinct separate ostia in the left sinus of Valsalva. Moreover, in <1% of the population, the LCX originates from a separate ostia in the right sinus of Valsalva or from the proximal RCA and usually courses posterior to the aorta to supply the lateral wall of the left ventricle (*Figure 3*).

Coronary Artery Anomalies Associated With Congenital Heart Diseases

Several anomalies of coronary origin have been well characterized. In tetralogy of Fallot, the LAD arises from the RCA or right sinus of Valsalva in approximately 10% of patients (*Figure 4*). This is of clinical relevance if any surgical procedure is planned on the right ventricular outflow tract (RVOT) because this LAD anomaly courses anteriorly across the RVOT to the anterior interventricular groove.

D-transposition of the great arteries (D-TGA) is characterized by the origin of the aorta from the right ventricle and the pulmonary artery from the left ventricle. The normal anatomic configuration with the pulmonary artery anterior to the aorta is lost in D-TGA. One way to describe the origin of the coronary arteries in patients with D-TGA is to imagine standing in the pulmonary artery facing the aorta. In this orientation, the right hand represents the right sinus of Valsalva and the left hand represents the left sinus of Valsalva (*Figure 5*). Approximately two-thirds of patients with D-TGA have an RCA that originates from the posterior sinus of Valsalva. Meanwhile, in approximately 20% of patients with D-TGA, both the RCA and LCX originate from the posterior sinus of Valsalva.

Anomalies of Coronary Course

Myocardial bridging occurs when a coronary artery, most commonly the LAD, descends from the epicardial course into the myocardium (*Video 1*). This is observed during diagnostic coronary angiography with some frequency. Likewise, this phenomenon is also reported with compression of proximal septal perforator branches in patients with hypertrophic cardiomyopathy. Because most coronary blood flow occurs during diastole, this is rarely of clinical importance.

 Video - not available for print.

Video 1

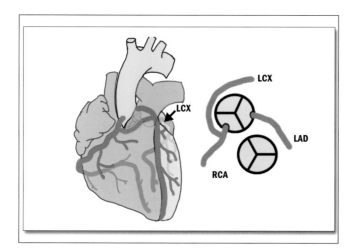

Figure 3a

Left Circumflex Coronary Artery Arising From the Right Coronary Artery

LAD = left anterior descending; LCX = left circumflex coronary; RCA = right coronary artery.

Image courtesy of Thomas Bashore, MD, ACCSAP 8.

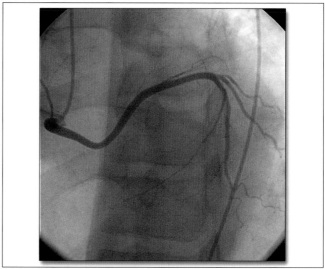

Figure 3b

Circumflex Coronary Artery From the Right Coronary Artery During Selective Coronary Angiography

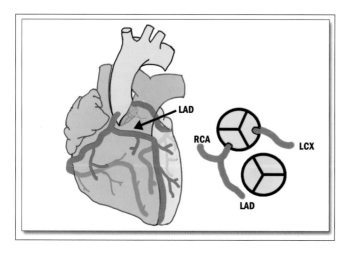

Figure 4

Anomalous Left Anterior Descending Artery Course in Tetralogy of Fallot

The LAD arises from the RCA and courses anterior to the right ventricular outflow tract.

LAD = left anterior descending; LCX = left circumflex; RCA = right coronary artery.

Image courtesy of Thomas Bashore, MD, ACCSAP 8.

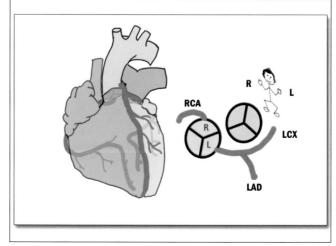

Figure 5

Coronary Anatomy in D-Transposition of the Great Arteries

L = left; LAD = left anterior descending; LCX = left circumflex; R = right; RCA = right coronary artery.

Image courtesy of Thomas Bashore, MD, ACCSAP 8.

- **Anomalies of Coronary Origin**
  - Anomalous coronary artery from the opposite sinus of Valsalva with course between aorta and pulmonary artery
  - Associated with supravalvular aortic stenosis
  - D-transposition of the great vessels following arterial switch procedure
  - Anomalous origin from the pulmonary artery (ALCAPA or ARCAPA)
  - Rarely, single coronary from right cusp
- **Anomalies of Coronary Course**
  - Myocardial bridging with documented ischemia
- **Anomalies of the Vessel Wall**
  - Congenital ostial stenosis
  - Coronary ectasia or aneurysm of large size
- **Anomalies of Coronary Destination**
  - Large coronary fistula

Table 2

Coronary Artery Anomalies With Potential Clinical Relevance

ALCAPA = anomalous left coronary artery from the pulmonary artery; ARCAPA = anomalous right coronary artery from the pulmonary artery.

Anomalies of the Vessel Wall

By definition, an aneurysm is a focal dilated segment of artery that is 1.5 times greater than the nearby reference normal vessel. This may be associated with coronary artery atherosclerosis, Kawasaki disease, or congenital disorders, such as Ehlers-Danlos syndrome. Diffuse regions of dilation may be present and are termed ectasia (*Video 2*). These are generally not associated with any clinical problems.

Video - not available for print.

Video 2

Anomalies of Coronary Destination

Coronary artery fistulas are rare, being reported in 0.1% of the population. Large fistulas are even more uncommon, with 225 reported from a large database of 126,000 catheterizations.[1] When present, coronary fistula often drain to low pressure, right-sided chambers, such as the right atrium, superior vena cava, coronary sinus, or pulmonary artery. Occasionally Thebesian veins are observed during diagnostic coronary angiography (*Video 3*). These are connections between the coronary veins and the left ventricle and create no potential clinical harm.

Video - not available for print.

Video 3

Key Point

- The most common coronary anomalies without clinical significance are separate origin of the right conus artery, separate ostia of the LAD and LCX, and origin of the LCX from the RCA or right sinus of Valsalva.

Coronary Anomalies with Potential Clinical Consequence

Table 2 describes coronary artery anomalies that may be associated with clinical sequela.

Anomalies of Coronary Origin

Anomalous coronary artery from the opposite sinus of Valsalva occurs when the LAD or left main originates from the right sinus of Valsalva or the RCA originates from the left sinus of Valsalva. This is a rare anomaly with one publication reporting 196 cases in a database of 126,595 catheterizations and another reporting 301 cases in a database of 210,700 catheterizations.[1,5] However, 4-14% of sudden cardiac deaths in college athletes were linked to an anomalous coronary from the opposite sinus of Valsalva.[6,7] When a coronary artery originates from the opposite sinus of Valsalva, it may take one of four possible courses: anterior to the pulmonary artery, posterior to the aorta, into the interventricular septum, or between the aorta and pulmonary artery (*Figure 6*).

It is only the variant with a course between the aorta and pulmonary artery that is associated with a sudden death risk, and it is quite statistically rare. A recent publication reported that only 54 of 210,700 catheterizations had an

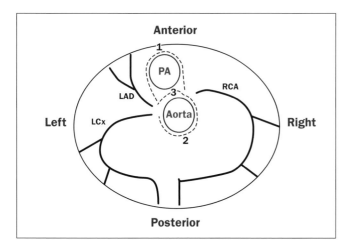

Figure 6

Potential Courses of an Anomalous Coronary Artery From the Opposite Sinus of Valsalva

Three subtypes of anomalous coronary artery from the opposite sinus of Valsalva.

1) Anterior course to the pulmonary artery (PA). 2) Posterior course to aorta. 3) Interarterial-between the aorta and PA.

LAD = left anterior descending; LCx = left circumflex; RCA = right coronary artery.

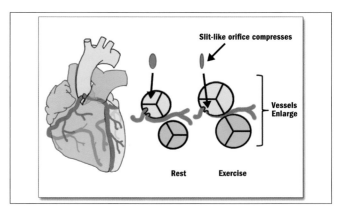

Figure 7

Postulated Etiology of Ischemia With Anomalous Coronary Artery From the Opposite Sinus of Valsalva

During exercise, the aorta and pulmonary artery dilate and the abnormal geometry of the anomalous coronary ostium is stretched further leading to reduced flow through the coronary ostium and subsequent ischemia.

Image courtesy of Thomas Bashore, MD, ACCSAP 8.

interarterial course of an anomalous coronary from the opposite sinus of Valsalva.

The mechanism leading to potential sudden death with an interarterial course of an anomalous coronary from the opposite sinus of Valsalva has been debated for years. Recent work from intravascular ultrasound studies supports a mechanism in which a slit-like orifice with abnormal geometry limits flow through the anomalous coronary during exercise (*Figure 7*).[8]

Defining the course of an anomalous coronary artery from the opposite sinus of Valsalva can be done in several ways. Historically, this was performed in the cardiac catheterization laboratory with simultaneous injection of the coronary and pulmonary artery in the 30° right anterior oblique and 60° left anterior oblique projections, with imaging continued into the levophase.[9] The current gold standard to define the anatomic course of an anomalous coronary from the opposite sinus is computed tomography (CT) angiography or cardiac magnetic resonance imaging (MRI). Imaging with CT or MRI is a Class I recommendation in the American College of Cardiology (ACC)/American Heart Association (AHA) 2008 Guidelines for the Management of Adults With Congenital Heart Disease.[10] The role for routine intravascular ultrasound evaluation of this anatomy at the time of catheterization has yet to be established and is not recommended for evaluation in the ACC/AHA 2008 Guidelines for the Management of Adults With Congenital Heart Disease.[10]

Recommendations for the management of patients with an anomalous coronary from the opposite sinus of Valsalva

have been published in the ACC/AHA 2008 Guidelines for the Management of Adults With Congenital Heart Disease.[10]

Class I recommendations include surgical revascularization in patients with:

- Anomalous left main coursing between the aorta and pulmonary artery.

- Anomalous coronary between the aorta and pulmonary artery and documented ischemia.

- Anomalous RCA coursing between the aorta and pulmonary artery with documented ischemia.

Class IIa recommendations state that surgical revascularization can be beneficial with established vascular wall hypoplasia, coronary compression, or obstruction to coronary blood flow, irrespective of documented ischemia.

Class IIb recommendations state that surgical revascularization may be reasonable when the LAD courses between the aorta and pulmonary artery.

Surgical revascularization for cases of an anomalous coronary artery from the opposite sinus of Valsalva commonly involves an unroofing procedure to create a neo-ostium (*Figure 8*). A recent retrospective analysis of patients with this anatomy who underwent surgical revascularization did not demonstrate any long-term survival benefit versus those who did not have surgery.[5]

Another anomaly of coronary artery origin occurs in patients with supravalvular aortic stenosis. Ostial coronary artery narrowing, coronary ectasia, or aneurysms may develop in supravalvular aortic stenosis. Periodic screening for myocardial ischemia is recommended in the ACC/

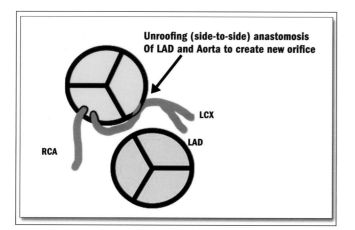

Figure 8

Surgical Repair of Anomalous Coronary From the Opposite Sinus of Valsalva

LAD = left anterior descending; LCX = left circumflex; RCA = right coronary artery.

Image courtesy of Thomas Bashore, MD, ACCSAP 8.

AHA 2008 Guidelines for the Management of Adults With Congenital Heart Disease.[10]

Anomalous Left Coronary Artery From the Pulmonary Artery

Anomalous left coronary artery from the pulmonary artery (ALCAPA), also known as Bland-Garland-White syndrome, is another anomaly of coronary origin with serious clinical implications (*Figure 9*; *Video 4*).[10] Usually this rare entity presents during infancy as congestive heart failure, but occasionally this is diagnosed in an adult patient if significant collaterals from the RCA to the LAD and LCX develop. The ACC/AHA 2008 Guidelines for the Management of Adults With Congenital Heart Disease suggest as a Class I recommendation surgical restoration of dual coronary circulation by a trained congenital cardiac surgeon.[10] In addition, noninvasive stress testing is recommended (Class I) every 3-5 years after surgical correction of ALCAPA.

Video - not available for print.

Video 4

Surgical Repair

For surgical repair, several approaches are used to correct this congenital anomaly:

- Ligation of the left coronary arising from the pulmonary artery with anastomosis of the left subclavian artery to the LAD has been reported in young children.

- Ligation of the coronary with saphenous vein or left internal mammary artery grafting to the LAD.

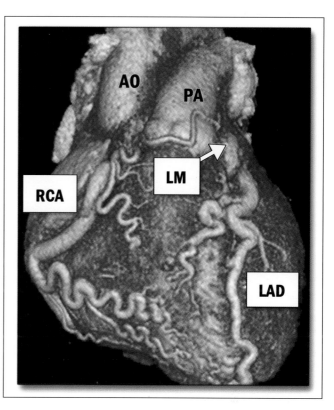

Figure 9

Anomalous Left Coronary Artery From the Pulmonary Artery

Computed tomography reconstruction demonstrating the origin of the LM from the PA. The RCA is dilated with significant collateral vessels to the LAD.

AO = aorta; LAD = left anterior descending; LM = left main; PA = pulmonary artery; RCA = right coronary artery.

Image courtesy of Thomas Bashore, MD, ACCSAP 8.

- Takeuchi procedure: an aortopulmonary window is created, and then a tunnel is constructed from the ostium of the anomalous coronary to the aorta traversing the pulmonary artery to perfuse the coronary.

- Anomalous coronary and a surrounding button of tissue are removed and reimplanted on the aorta.

Anomalous Right Coronary Artery From the Pulmonary Artery

Even less common than ALCAPA is an anomalous right coronary artery from the pulmonary artery (*Figures 10, 11; Video 5*). There are just over 100 cases reported in the literature. Perfusion of the normal RCA myocardial territory is dependent on collateral formation from the left coronary circulation. Management involves surgical reimplantation of the RCA on the aorta.

Video - not available for print.

Video 5

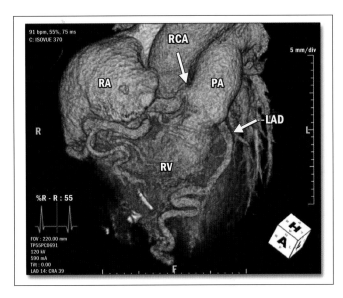

Figure 10
Anomalous Right Coronary Artery From the Pulmonary Artery

Computed tomography reconstruction demonstrating the origin of the RCA from the PA. The LAD is dilated with significant collateral vessels to the RCA.

LAD = left anterior descending; PA = pulmonary artery; RA = right atrium; RCA = right coronary artery; RV = right ventricle.

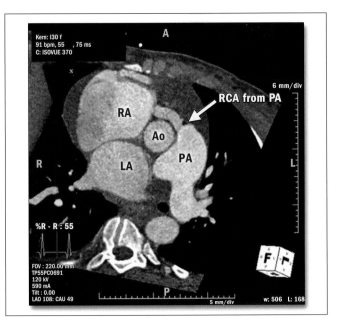

Figure 11
Axial Computed Tomography Image Demonstrating the Origin of the Right Coronary Artery From the Pulmonary Artery

Ao = aorta; LA = left atrium; PA = pulmonary artery; RA = right atrium; RCA = right coronary artery.

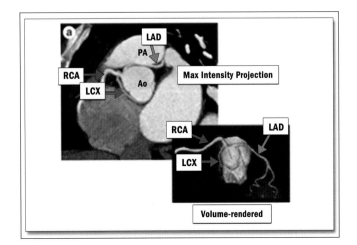

Figure 12
Anomalous Origin of All Three Coronaries From the Right Sinus of Valsalva

The computed tomography imaging demonstrates the course of the LAD between the Ao and PA. The LCX originates from the proximal RCA and courses posterior to the Ao.

Ao = aorta; LAD = left anterior descending; LCX = left circumflex; PA = pulmonary artery; RCA = right coronary artery.

Image courtesy of Thomas Bashore, MD, ACCSAP 8.

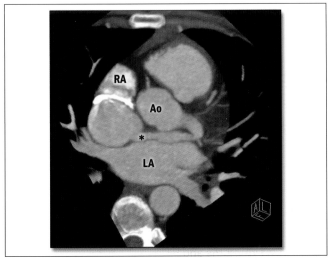

Figure 13
Large Coronary Fistula From the Left Main to the Right Atrium

Axial oblique computed tomography imaging demonstrating the origin of the fistula from the left main coursing posterior to the Ao to empty into the RA. The asterisk (*) represents the coronary fistula.

Ao = aorta; LA = left atrium; RA = right atrium.

Reproduced with permission from Kiefer TL, Vavalle J, Halim S, et al. Anterograde percutaneous coronary-cameral fistula closure employing a guide-in-guide technique. JACC Cardiovasc Interv 2013;6:1105-7.

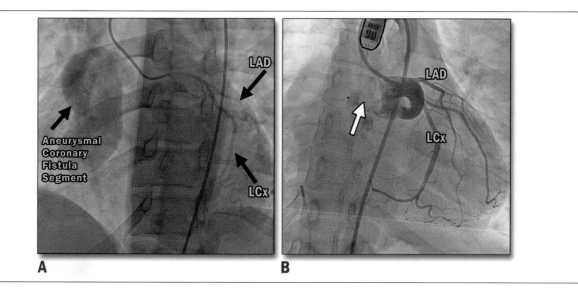

Figure 14

Angiography of a Large Coronary Fistula to the Right Atrium Before and After Closure With an Amplatzer Vascular Plug II

Coronary angiography demonstrating a large coronary fistula draining into a large aneurysmal segment and then into the right atrium before (panel A) and after (panel B) successful percutaneous closure with an AMPLATZER Vascular Plug II. The white arrow in panel B is the 12 mm AMPLATZER Vascular Plug II.

LAD = left anterior descending; LCx = left circumflex coronary artery.

Reproduced with permission from Kiefer TL, Vavalle J, Halim S, et al. Anterograde percutaneous coronary-camera fistula closure employing a guide-in-guide technique. JACC Cardiovasc Interv 2013;6:1105-7.

Single Coronary

Single coronary is an extremely rare finding that has been associated with sudden cardiac death (*Figure 12*; *Video 6*). The adult congenital guidelines do not address management of this anomaly.

Video - not available for print.

Video 6

Anomalies of Coronary Course

Most coronary muscle bridges are asymptomatic. Infrequently, symptoms and ischemia may be documented with this anomaly. In cases of documented ischemia in symptomatic patients without other etiology and refractory to medical therapy, surgical unroofing or bypass grafting may be considered.

Anomalies of the Vessel Wall

Anomalies of the vessel wall include severe ectasia, large aneurysms, or ostial stenosis. In most cases, ectasia and large aneurysms are associated with coronary atherosclerotic disease rather than Kawasaki disease. Thrombotic events leading to coronary occlusion have been reported in the literature.

There is a paucity of data or guidelines for the management of these anomalies. Surgical resection and covered stent placement across an aneurysm have both been published in the literature.[11] In addition, use of antiplatelet and anticoagulant therapy has also been anecdotally reported in the literature.

Anomalies of Coronary Destination

As previously described in this review, large coronary fistulas are quite uncommon. However, there are cases in which a large coronary fistula develops, leading to volume loading of the receiving chamber from a shunt of significant magnitude, arrhythmias, and/or coronary steal. Imaging with CT or MRI is informative to understand the route and sites of fistula insertion (*Figure 13*). Surgical and percutaneous approaches to closure have been reported (*Figure 14; Video 7*).[12]

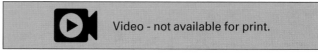
Video - not available for print.

Video 7

The ACC/AHA 2008 Guidelines for the Management of Adults With Congenital Heart Disease[10] suggest the following as Class I recommendations:

- Large fistulas, even in asymptomatic patients, should be closed either via transcatheter or a surgical approach.

- Small or moderate fistulas should be closed if there is documented ischemia, arrhythmias, or systolic or diastolic dysfunction without other etiology, chamber enlargement, or in rare cases of endarteritis.

Key Points

- The most important coronary anomaly of potential clinical significance is anomalous coronary artery from the opposite sinus of Valsalva. It is rare, being observed in 0.1% of cardiac catheterizations. This anomaly may be the RCA from the left sinus of Valsalva or the left main or LAD from the right sinus of Valsalva. Studies of sudden death in college athletes have reported that 4-14% of events are attributable to an anomalous coronary artery from the opposite sinus of Valsalva. The mechanism of sudden death seems to be related to decreased blood flow, leading to myocardial ischemia from an abnormal slit-like orifice of the anomalous coronary ostium. Surgical unroofing is recommended in cases of the left main or LAD from the right sinus of Valsalva with or without documented ischemia or the RCA from the left sinus of Valsalva with documented ischemia.

- Large coronary fistulae are exceedingly rare. Closure should be considered in cases of congestive heart failure related to the fistulae, arrhythmias, chamber enlargement, or coronary steal.

Conclusions

There are a variety of coronary anomalies. Most are quite rare and do not lead to clinical sequela. However, understanding which anomalies have potentially serious complications and the appropriate evaluation and management strategies is important for cardiovascular practitioners.

References

1. Yamanaka O, Hobbs RE. Coronary artery anomalies in 126,595 patients undergoing coronary arteriography. Cathet Cardiovasc Diagn 1990;21:28-40.

2. Ogden JA. Congenital anomalies of the coronary arteries. Am J Cardiol 1970;25:474-9.

3. Angelini P. Coronary artery anomalies--current clinical issues: definitions, classification, incidence, clinical relevance, and treatment guidelines. Tex Heart Inst J 2002;29:271-8.

4. Jacobs ML, Mavroudis C. Anomalies of the coronary arteries: nomenclature and classification. Cardiol Young 2010;20 Suppl 3:15-9.

5. Krasuski RA, Magyar D, Hart S, et al. Long-term outcome and impact of surgery on adults with coronary arteries originating from the opposite coronary cusp. Circulation 2011;123:154-62.

6. Maron BJ. Sudden death in young athletes. N Engl J Med 2003;349:1064-75.

7. Maron BJ, Haas TS, Murphy CJ, Ahluwalia A, Rutten-Ramos S. Incidence and causes of sudden death in U.S. college athletes. J Am Coll Cardiol 2014;63:1636-43.

8. Angelini P, Velasco JA, Flamm S. Coronary anomalies: incidence, pathophysiology, and clinical relevance. Circulation 2002;105:2449-54.

9. Wang A, Pulsipher MW, Jaggers J, et al. Simultaneous biplane coronary and pulmonary arteriography: a novel technique for defining the course of an anomalous left main coronary artery originating from the right sinus of Valsalva. Cathet Cardiovasc Diagn 1997;42:73-8.

10. Warnes CA, Williams RG, Bashore TM, et al. ACC/AHA 2008 guidelines for the management of adults with congenital heart disease: a report of the American College of Cardiology/American Heart Association Task Force on Practice Guidelines (Writing Committee to Develop Guidelines on the Management of Adults With Congenital Heart Disease). Developed in Collaboration With the American Society of Echocardiography, Heart Rhythm Society, International Society for Adult Congenital Heart Disease, Society for Cardiovascular Angiography and Interventions, and Society of Thoracic Surgeons. J Am Coll Cardiol 2008;52:e143-263.

11. Ferlini M, Russo F, Marinoni B, et al. Images in cardiology. Percutaneous coronary aneurysm obliteration using a novel pericardium-covered stent. J Am Coll Cardiol 2010;56:2139.

12. Kiefer TL, Vavalle J, Halim S, et al. Anterograde percutaneous coronary-cameral fistula closure employing a guide-in-guide technique. JACC Cardiovasc Interv 2013;6:1105-7.

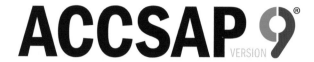

ACCSAP 9 VERSION ®

Adult Clinical Cardiology Self-Assessment Program

Book
Vascular Diseases

DISEASES OF THE AORTA

Editor:
Patrick T. O'Gara, MD, MACC
This author has nothing to disclose.

Aortic Aneurysm Disease

Introduction

A true aneurysm is a permanent localized dilatation of an artery, having at least a 50% increase in diameter (i.e., ≥1.5 times larger) compared with the expected normal diameter. Although by definition all three histologic layers of the artery (intima, media, adventitia) are present, the intima and media in large aneurysms may be significantly attenuated.

A thoracic aortic aneurysm (TAA) may involve the aortic root, ascending aorta, aortic arch, or the descending aorta above the diaphragm. The aneurysm may involve one or more segments. When the aneurysm involves the thoracic and abdominal aorta, it is referred to as a thoracoabdominal aneurysm.

Thoracic Aortic Aneurysm Disease

The thoracic aorta is divided into four parts: 1) aortic root, including the aortic valve annulus, the aortic valve cusps, and the sinuses of Valsalva; 2) ascending aorta, including the tubular portion of the ascending aorta beginning at the sinotubular junction and extending to the brachiocephalic artery origin; 3) aortic arch, starting at the origin of the brachiocephalic artery, and including the origin of the head and neck arteries, coursing anterior to both trachea and esophagus; and 4) descending aorta, starting at the isthmus between the origin of the left subclavian artery and the ligamentum arteriosum and coursing anterior to the vertebral column, and then through the diaphragm into the abdomen.

Etiology

The most common etiologies of TAA disease are listed in *Table 1*. Among patients with an aneurysm in one segment of the aorta, there is a 25% chance of having a concomitant aneurysm involving another aortic segment. Aneurysms that involve the aortic root and ascending aorta are encountered most commonly, and usually occur as a consequence of underlying medial degeneration, a process that includes loss of smooth muscle cells, elastic fiber fragmentation, and increased deposition of proteoglycans. These changes result in weakening of the tensile strength of the aortic wall. Recent literature supports the presence of inflammatory cells in this condition.[1,2]

Ascending aortic aneurysms may be idiopathic, but in many such cases histologic analysis will reveal medial degeneration. In aneurysms that occur sporadically, other family members may be affected in about 20% of cases. Several genetic conditions are associated with the development of TAAs, including Marfan syndrome (MFS), Loeys-Dietz syndrome, Turner syndrome, bicuspid aortic valve (BAV) disease, and familial thoracic aortic aneurysm disease (FTAAD) (*Table 1*).

Aortic aneurysms also occur in association with mutations of myosin heavy chain 11 (*MYH11*) and actin/alpha 2 (*ACTA2*) genes, leading to aortic smooth muscle cell hyperplasia and ascending aortic aneurysms. The aortic media in aneurysm tissue taken from patients with mutations in these genes demonstrates focal hyperplasia associated with smooth muscle cells that show a lack of structured orientation.[3,4]

Prashanth Vallabhajosyula, MD, MS
This author has nothing to disclose.

Andreas Habertheuer, MD
This author has nothing to disclose.

Joseph E. Bavaria, MD, FACC
Consultant Fees/Honoraria: St. Jude Medical; Research/Research Grants: Boston Scientific, Edwards Lifesciences, Medtronic, Vascutek, W.L. Gore & Associates.

Learner Objectives

Upon completion of this module, the reader will be able to:

1. Recognize both acquired and genetic causes of thoracic aortic aneurysm (TAA) and abdominal aortic aneurysm (AAA) disease.
2. Apply guideline recommendations for the clinical and imaging assessment of aortic aneurysm disease using ultrasonography, computed tomography (CT), and magnetic resonance (MR) imaging.
3. Incorporate current recommendations for medical management of aortic aneurysm disease.
4. Apply recommendations for referral for surgical or endovascular repair.
5. Appreciate outcomes of surgical and endovascular therapy for aortic aneurysm disease.
6. Apply current recommendations for screening at-risk individuals for aortic aneurysm disease.

Atherosclerosis
(Typically affects the descending aorta.)
Hypertension
(Typically affects the ascending aorta.)
Connective Tissue Disease
(Typically affects the ascending aorta.)
○ Marfan syndrome (*FBN-1* mutations)
○ Vascular Ehlers-Danlos type IV (*COL3A1* mutations)
○ Loeys-Dietz syndrome (TGF-beta receptor 1 or 2 mutations)
○ Turner syndrome (XO syndrome)
○ Bicuspid aortic valve disease (no single mutation)
○ Familial thoracic aortic aneurysm disease (several mutations)
Inflammatory Diseases
○ Giant cell arteritis
○ Takayasu arteritis
○ Psoriatic aortitis
○ Inflammatory bowel disease
○ Behcet's disease
○ Reiter's syndrome
○ Ankylosing spondylitis (HLA-B27)
○ Sarcoidosis
Infectious Acquired Causes
○ Syphilis (treponema pallidum)
○ Mycobacterium tuberculosis
Traumatic Aortic Injury (Transection with Pseudo-Aneurysm)
Chronic Aortic Dissection (False Lumen Enlargement)

Table 1

Etiologies of Thoracic Aortic Aneurysm Disease

The role of genetic testing in patients with TAAs remains to be clarified. Nevertheless, given the fact that aneurysm disease can be inherited, first-degree relatives of selected individuals should be screened for thoracic aortic disease with diagnostic imaging. The role of routine echocardiographic screening of first-degree relatives of patients with BAV disease (with or without aortopathy) is controversial. BAV disease affects up to 1.5% of the general population, thus screening programs would be large and expensive, with relatively little yield. Some advocate that a carefully performed physical examination should be the first screening tool in first-degree family members of patients with BAV disease.

Medial degeneration is well recognized in MFS, a connective tissue disorder associated with decreased elastin in the aortic media. MFS is an autosomal dominant disorder which affects cardiac, vascular, ocular, and bony structures, and is due to mutations in the *FBN-1* gene, which encodes fibrillin-1. Apart from its structural importance, fibrillin-1 also plays a role in regulating transforming growth factor (TGF)-β pathways. In MFS, there is excessive TGF-β signaling, which in turn leads to elastin fiber fragmentation and progressive aortic root enlargement and the clinical sequelae of aneurysm, dissection, and rupture.

In a mouse model of MFS, treatment with a TGF-β neutralizing antibody reduced TGF-β signaling in the aortic media and arrested aortic growth.[5] The angiotensin-receptor blocker losartan inhibits TGF-β signaling in a similar fashion.[5] Clinical trials in humans, however, have been disappointing. Specifically, in children and young adults with MFS, there was no difference in the rate of growth of the aortic root with losartan compared with atenolol.[6]

BAV is the most common congenital valve disorder (prevalence 1-1.5% of the general population, with a 4:1 male predominance), and is an important risk factor for aortic root and ascending aortic aneurysm development.

Approximately 50% of patients with BAV have enlargement of the proximal aorta, independent of the function of the aortic valve. Aortic dilatation occurs with equal incidence in patients with normally functioning bicuspid valves, aortic regurgitation, or aortic stenosis. Moreover, among BAV patients undergoing aortic valve replacement surgery for aortic stenosis, 75% are found to have medial degeneration compared with only 14% of patients with trileaflet aortic stenosis.

Aortic aneurysm disease occurs in several inflammatory syndromes, including giant cell arteritis (usually affecting older woman and often with polymyalgia rheumatica), Takayasu arteritis (affecting younger women with left subclavian artery involvement), psoriasis, inflammatory bowel disease, Behcet's disease, Reiter's syndrome, ankylosing spondylitis (HLA-B27), and sarcoidosis. Infectious causes include syphilis and tuberculosis. While hypertension is associated with TAA disease, atherosclerosis is more commonly associated with both descending TAA and AAA disease.

Natural History
Most TAAs grow over time. The rate of growth is greater for large versus small aneurysms, as predicted by the Laplace relation, in patients with MFS, in patients with chronic aortic dissection, and in patients with aneurysms involving the descending, rather than the ascending, aorta. The risk of rupture increases significantly at diameters ≥6 cm.

1. Asymptomatic Ascending	
a. Degenerative	≥5.5 cm
b. Genetic syndrome	4.0-5.0 cm depending on specific condition and family history
c. BAV	≥5.5 cm >5.0 cm if additional risk factor for dissection present >4.5 cm at time of operation for severe valve disease
2. Symptomatic TAA	any size
3. Asymptomatic Arch	>5.5 cm (low-risk patient)
4. Asymptomatic Descending	>5.5 cm (low-risk patient) >6.0 cm (high-risk patient, no TEVAR option)

Table 2

Recommendations for Surgery for TAA Disease Based on Size and Rate of Growth of Aneurysm

BAV = bicuspid aortic valve; TAA = thoracic aortic aneurysm; TEVAR = thoracic endovascular aortic repair.

Presentation

Most TAAs are asymptomatic and not detectable on routine physical examination. The large majority are discovered incidentally on an imaging study ordered for another indication. Root and ascending aortic aneurysms may result in malcoaptation of the aortic valve leaflets and functional aortic regurgitation. Aortic regurgitation may present early, as a diastolic heart murmur, or late, with heart failure. Less often, thoracic aneurysms present with symptoms caused by a mass effect, such as cough, dysphagia, or hoarseness due to tracheal, esophageal, or recurrent laryngeal nerve compression, respectively.

Assessment

TAAs can be detected by CT angiography (CTA), MR angiography (MRA), echocardiography, and aortography. CTA is used most often for evaluation of the thoracic aorta, as it provides outstanding anatomic detail and accurate sizing of the aorta. MRA also images the aorta well, although it is less convenient and cannot be used in patients with implanted cardiac devices.

Transthoracic echocardiography provides excellent visualization of the aortic root, but is less reliable in imaging the ascending aorta. Transesophageal echocardiography images the thoracic aorta well, but not completely. Invasive aortography can identify dilated aortic segments, but cannot be used to size the aorta accurately and may miss other pathologies (e.g., intramural hematoma). Although once regarded as the gold standard, invasive aortography is no longer the imaging test of first choice. CT angiography is most commonly utilized.

Treatment and Surveillance

Medical Treatment of Thoracic Aortic Aneurysm Disease

The goal of medical therapy is to reduce aortic wall stress by controlling heart rate (≤60 bpm) and blood pressure (target systolic blood pressure 110-120 mm Hg). Beta-blockers have long been the mainstay of medical therapy for TAAs. They should be used cautiously in patients with severe aortic regurgitation. In patients with pulmonary contraindications to beta-blockers (e.g., asthma), a nondihydropyridine calcium-channel blocker is recommended.

After adequate heart rate control has been achieved, an angiotensin-converting enzyme inhibitor or other vasodilator may be used if the blood pressure remains above 120 mm Hg. Vasodilating beta-blockers (e.g., carvedilol) may be effective. Statin and aspirin therapy should be provided according to current guideline recommendations. The presence of aortic atherosclerosis (the most common cause of descending thoracic aortic aneurysms) is indicative of established cardiovascular disease for which aggressive treatment is warranted.

Surveillance imaging is required to monitor aortic growth. In most cases, the imaging should be repeated annually, but especially when the maximal aortic diameter begins to approach the lower size threshold for elective repair. Once this occurs, patients also should be referred to an appropriate aortic specialist for evaluation. Patients with confirmed genetic mutations predisposing to TAA and dissection (MFS with *FBN-1 mutation*, Loeys-Dietz syndrome with *TGFRB1, TGFRB2 mutations, ACTA1,* and *MYH11 mutations*) should undergo complete aortic imaging at diagnosis and 6 months thereafter to assess for enlargement. Patients with Loeys-Dietz syndrome should additionally undergo extended vascular imaging from the head to the pelvis.

Surgical Treatment of Thoracic Aortic Aneurysm Disease

Mortality associated with aortic dissection or rupture is high, whereas the mortality of an elective repair is reasonably low. The goal is to repair the at-risk aorta prior to any catastrophic event. Indications for repair of asymptomatic TAAs are reviewed in the 2010 guideline for

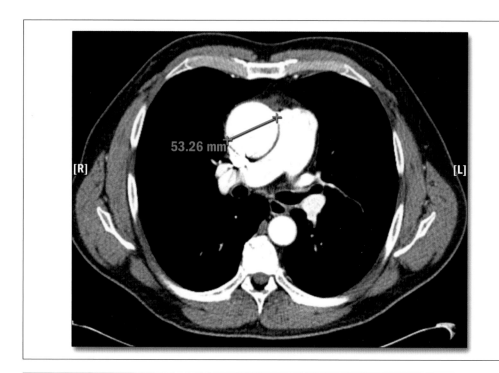

Figure 1
Isolated Ascending Aortic Aneurysm

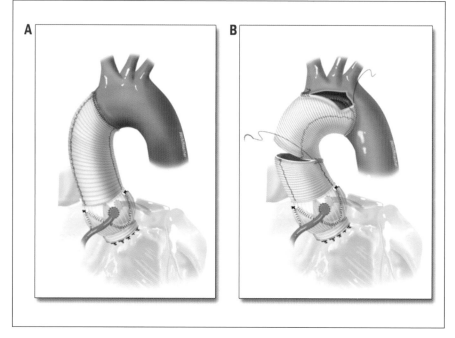

Figure 2
The David Procedure

Illustration of the valve-sparing root reimplantation procedure (David) with replacement of the ascending aorta (**panel A**) and aggressive hemiarch (**panel B**). After cross clamp is applied on heart-lung bypass, the aorta is incised just above the origins of the coronary arteries for exposure of the aortic root. The coronary arteries are detached from the root in common fashion with buttons of surrounding tissue. The sinuses are then removed, leaving behind the native valve. After measuring the valve size, a graft of appropriate size is sutured into the aortic root. The graft is slightly over the aortic root and the valve is brought inside. Sutures are placed on each commissure to resuspend the native valve in the tube graft. The procedure is completed with reimplantation of the coronary buttons and distal anastomosis of the distal ascending aorta (**panel A**) or hemiarch (**panel B**).

Courtesy of Wilson Y. Szeto, MD. Penn Medicine, Philadelphia, PA.

the diagnosis and management of patients with thoracic aortic disease[7] and its 2016 update.[8] All symptomatic TAAs should be urgently evaluated for immediate intervention (*Table 2*).

Open repair is required for aneurysms involving the root and ascending aorta. If the ascending aorta alone is enlarged (*Figure 1*), a simple interposition tube graft should suffice. If the aortic root is enlarged, two traditional procedures are available. The Bentall procedure involves replacement of the aortic valve and root using a composite valve-graft conduit and reimplantation of the coronary arteries. If the aortic valve leaflets are healthy, the native valve can be preserved and resuspended within a prosthetic tube graft, in what is known as valve-sparing root reimplantation or David procedure (*Figure 2*). The David procedure is more complex than the Bentall procedure, and it is recommended that it be performed at high-volume centers of excellence.

When the aortic arch is significantly dilated, a total arch replacement is usually required. Most often this is performed using a multibranched prosthetic arch graft, to which each arch vessel is connected individually.

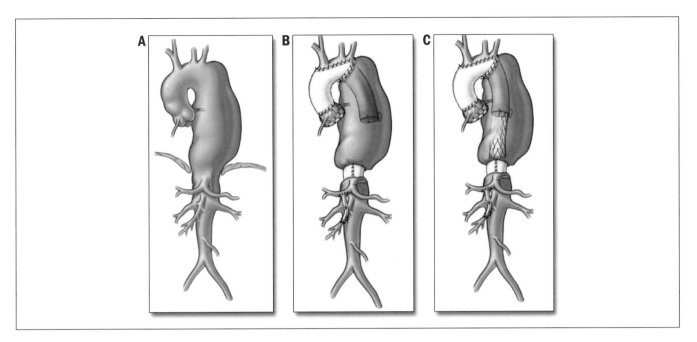

Figure 3
Elephant Trunk Procedure

Panel A: Preoperative stage. Thoracoabdominal aneurysm extending well beyond the level of the renal arteries, without involvement of the aortic root. **Panel B**: Stage 1 of procedure. Supracoronary replacement of the ascending aorta and transverse arch with a polyester fiber graft (i.e., Dacron) prosthesis and islet patch reimplantation of the supra-aortic large vessels. The distal end of the Dacron graft is sutured circumferentially to the distal transverse/proximal descending aorta, with the free floating end of the distal graft within the descending aorta. Variants of this procedure have been described. In this case, a prosthesis is interposed in the descending abdominal aorta. **Panel C**: Stage 2 of procedure. After a variable interval, an endovascular stent graft is attached proximally to the free floating elephant trunk and distally to the abdominal prosthesis cuff.

Reproduced with permission from Hiratzka LF, Bakris GL, Beckman JA, et al. 2010 ACCF/AHA/AATS/ACR/ASA/SCA/SCAI/SIR/STS/SVM guidelines for the diagnosis and management of patients with thoracic aortic disease. A report of the American College of Cardiology Foundation/American Heart Association Task Force on Practice Guidelines, American Association for Thoracic Surgery, American College of Radiology, American Stroke Association, Society of Cardiovascular Anesthesiologists, Society for Cardiovascular Angiography and Interventions, Society of Interventional Radiology, Society of Thoracic Surgeons, and Society for Vascular Medicine. J Am Coll Cardiol 2010;55:e27-e129.

Alternatively, all three arch vessels can be excised together as an islet patch. This approach is associated with shorter operative and ischemic times.

Neurological complications are the most frequently observed adverse events accompanying arch repair (either from hypoxia or central embolization of debris during surgery). Arch reconstruction requires circulatory arrest. Methods of cerebral protection include deep hypothermic circulatory arrest and antegrade and retrograde cerebral perfusion strategies.

Patients with very extensive aortic disease (i.e., aneurysms extending from the ascending aorta via the arch to the descending or thoracoabdominal aorta) might be offered a two-stage hybrid elephant trunk procedure (*Figure 3*). Although variations exist, the goal of the first stage of the procedure is to repair the proximal pathology (root, aortic valve, ascending aorta, transverse arch) with a tube graft. The distal end of the graft is sutured circumferentially to the aorta, distal to the left subclavian artery, and the free end of the graft (elephant trunk) floats freely within the descending

thoracic aorta. During the second stage of the procedure, an endovascular stent graft is attached proximally to the elephant trunk and distally to either healthy aortic tissue or an interposed tube graft in the descending thoracic aorta.

Endovascular Treatment of Thoracic Aortic Aneurysm Disease
Aneurysms of the descending thoracic aorta (*Figure 4*) have traditionally been repaired with open surgery via a left thoracotomy, a procedure historically associated with significant morbidity and mortality rates of up to 10%. The most feared complication is postoperative paraplegia from spinal cord ischemia. In recent years, thoracic endovascular aortic repair (TEVAR) with stent grafting has emerged as an alternative to open surgical repair for aneurysms of the descending thoracic aorta and is now considered the gold standard.

In a multicenter, prospective, nonrandomized, phase 2 study, TEVAR implantation was successful in 98% of patients, with 30-day event rates of 3% for paraplegia and 2% for death, significantly better than the respective event rates in an open surgical control population.[9] Even at 5

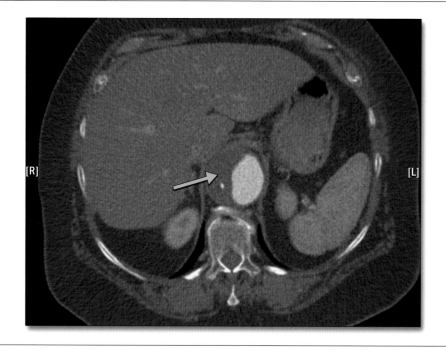

Figure 4
Aortic Aneurysm at the Level of the Diaphragm Consistent With Thoraco-Abdominal Location

Arrow points to intramural thrombus.

years, aneurysm-related mortality was lower for the TEVAR patients than for open controls (3% vs. 12%, respectively).[10] Despite this advantage, there was no difference in all-cause mortality at 5 years, likely reflecting the fact that the TEVAR patient population tends to be older and have multiple comorbidities, including coronary heart disease.

Key Points

- Inherited causes of TAA disease include Marfan Syndrome (*Fibrillin-1*), Loeys-Dietz syndrome (*TGFBR1/TGFBR2*), Ehlers-Danlos (*COL3A*) and Familial Thoracic Aortic Aneurysm Disease, among others. First-degree relatives of affected individuals should be screened.

- Medical therapy for TAA disease includes beta-blockade and the use of a vasodilating agent (such as an ACEI or ARB) if blood pressure remains elevated. Losartan did not prove more effective than atenolol for slowing the rate of aortic root enlargement in young patients with MFS. Statin and aspirin therapy should be provided according to current guideline recommendations for patients with atherosclerotic disease.

- Thoracic aortic disease is usually asymptomatic and detected on imaging performed for another indication.

- Recommendations for surgery for TAA disease depend on aneurysm size, its rate of growth, and the clinical context in which it is encountered (See *Table 2*).

Abdominal Aortic Aneurysm Disease

Although the normal diameter of the aorta varies with age, sex, and body habitus, the average diameter of the human infrarenal aorta is about 2.0 cm. The upper limit is typically <3.0 cm. An abdominal aorta with a maximal diameter >3.0 cm is considered aneurysmal in most adult patients. AAAs most often affect the segment of aorta between the renal and inferior mesenteric arteries (infrarenal). Approximately 5% of AAAs involve the renal or visceral arteries. Stagnation of blood flow may result in thrombus formation along the aneurysm wall. The thrombus may embolize distally, and its presence may increase the risk for aneurysm growth and rupture.[11]

Etiology, Risk Factors, and Pathogenesis

Atherosclerosis is the leading cause of aneurysm formation affecting the abdominal aorta. Age, male sex, smoking, family history, hypertension, and hyperlipidemia are the most common risk factors for AAAs, and are detailed in *Table 3*. AAAs are less commonly found in women (who nevertheless tend to rupture at smaller aortic diameters compared with men), African Americans, and patients with diabetes.

There is evidence that genetic, environmental, hemodynamic, inflammatory, and immunological factors also contribute to the development of AAAs.

Certain matrix metalloproteinases (MMPs), enzymes produced by smooth muscle and inflammatory cells, can degrade elastin and collagen, which in turn are the primary components of the aortic extracellular matrix. High levels of MMPs have been linked to aneurysm formation and growth.

In an animal model of AAA, treatment with doxycycline, which inhibits MMPs through a mechanism unrelated to its antibiotic activity, leads to lower levels of MMP-9 activity in the aortic wall and reduces expansion of aneurysms.[12] Early data from human trials have shown promising results, but randomized clinical trials have yet to be performed, and the use of such therapies is not currently recommended. Statin therapy has also been shown to reduce MMP-9 expression and to protect against aneurysm growth in the mouse model, regardless of the cholesterol level.[13] Additionally, in humans undergoing elective AAA repair, preoperative statin therapy is associated with a decrease in MMP-9 levels in the aortic wall.[14] Preoperative statin therapy is also associated with a reduction in the risk of perioperative ischemic events in patients undergoing various types of surgery for peripheral arterial disease.

Natural History

The true prevalence of AAA disease is not well known, due to variations in both diagnostic criteria and the baseline risk of the population screened. However, AAA is uncommon in people under the age of 60 years. About 0.1% of the general population develops an AAA between the ages of 60 and 65 years, and this percentage of affected individuals in the population continues to increase with age. Screening studies show that AAA occurs in up to 13% of men and 6% of women over the age of 65 years.

Presentation

Potential clinical manifestations of AAA disease are presented in *Table 4*.

Assessment

Most patients with AAAs are asymptomatic and their aneurysms are discovered incidentally on physical examination or on abdominal imaging ordered for another indication. Patients with symptoms usually present with

○ Smoking
○ Male sex *(but women rupture at smaller diameters)*
○ Age
○ Family history
○ Hypertension
○ Hyperlipidemia

Table 3
Risk Factors for Abdominal Aortic Aneurysms

pain in the hypogastrium or lower back. Aneurysm rupture is associated with the abrupt onset of pain. A tender, pulsatile abdominal mass is an ominous finding.

Several imaging techniques can identify and size AAAs. Abdominal ultrasonography is accepted as the most practical way to screen for AAAs, and to follow their size over time. This technique is inexpensive and without risk, but is limited in the accuracy of its measurements and in its ability to image the suprarenal aorta and branch vessels. CTA is very accurate in imaging and sizing all segments of the aorta, and in defining branch vessel anatomy. However, CTA is more expensive than ultrasonography and requires the use of iodinated contrast and exposure to radiation.

MRA can also provide accurate delineation of the abdominal aorta and its major branches. Contrast studies involve the use of gadolinium, which is contraindicated in patients with moderate or greater renal impairment. MRA is more sensitive than CTA for detection of endoleaks after EVAR. Compared with CTA, MRA is more expensive and less comfortable for some patients.

Pathophysiology	Related Clinical Manifestations
Compression of adjacent structures	Abdominal pain
	Chronic flank or back pain, vertebral effacement
	Ureteral obstruction and hydronephrosis
Acute or subacute symptoms caused by change in aneurysm size with inflammation and thrombosis	Localized dissection or intramural hematoma
	Aorto-enteric (usually duodenal) fistula with gastrointestinal bleeding
	Contained retroperitoneal rupture
	Distal arterial embolism of aneurysmal thrombus
Peritoneal free rupture	Hypotension
	Lactic acidosis
	Disseminated intravascular coagulation
	Shock
	Death

Table 4
Possible Clinical Manifestation of Abdominal Aortic Aneurysm Disease

Population	Men aged 65 to 75 y who have ever smoked*	Men aged 65 to 75 y who have never smoked	Women aged 65 to 75 y who have ever smoked*	Women who have never smoked
Recommendation	Screen once for abdominal aortic aneurysm (AAA) by ultrasonography. Grade: B	Selectively screen for AAA. Grade: C	No recommendation. Grade: I statement	Do not screen for AAA. Grade: D
Risk Assessment	Risk factors for AAA include older age; a positive smoking history; having a first-degree relative with an AAA; and having a history of other vascular aneurysms, coronary artery disease, cerebrovascular disease, atherosclerosis, hypercholesterolemia, obesity, or hypertension. Factors associated with a reduced risk for AAA include African American race, Hispanic ethnicity, and diabetes.			
Screening Tests	Abdominal duplex ultrasonography is the standard approach for AAA screening. Screening with ultrasonography is noninvasive and easy to perform and has high sensitivity (94% to 100%) and specificity (98% to 100%) for detection.			
Treatment	Patients with large AAAs (≥5.5 cm) are referred for open surgical repair or endovascular aneurysm repair. Patients with smaller aneurysms (3.0 to 5.4 cm) are generally managed conservatively via surveillance (e.g., repeated ultrasonography every 3 to 12 mo). Early open surgery for the treatment of smaller AAAs does not reduce AAA-specific or all-cause mortality. Surgical referral of smaller AAAs is typically reserved for rapid growth (>1.0 cm per year) or once the threshold of ≥5.5 cm on repeated ultrasonography is reached. Short-term treatment with antibiotics or β-blockers does not seem to reduce AAA growth.			
Balance of Benefits and Harms	There is a moderate net benefit of screening for AAA with ultrasonography in men aged 65 to 75 y who have ever smoked.	There is a small net benefit of screening for AAA with ultrasonography in men aged 65 to 75 y who have never smoked.	The evidence of screening for AAA in women aged 65 to 75 y who have ever smoked is insufficient, and the balance of benefits and harms cannot be determined.	The harms of screening for AAA in women who have never smoked outweigh any potential benefits.

Table 5

Recommendations for Screening for Abdominal Aortic Aneurysm From the U.S. Preventive Services Task Force

* "Ever smoked" is defined as having smoked at least 100 cigarettes during a lifetime.

Reproduced with permission from LeFevre ML, on behalf of the U.S. Preventive Services Task Force. Screening for abdominal aortic aneurysm: U.S. Preventive Services Task Force recommendation statement. Ann Intern Med 2014;161:281-90.

The US Preventive Services Task Force recommends ultrasonography screening for AAA disease one time in men ≥65 years who are current or previous smokers.[15] The full recommendations are presented in *Table 5*.

Medical Treatment

Patients who are not operated immediately or those who are awaiting intervention are followed carefully. The mainstays of medical management include aspirin and statin therapy for primary or secondary prevention, blood pressure control, and smoking cessation. At least one clinical study showed that beta-blockers reduced the rate of growth of AAAs compared with placebo, but their effectiveness has been questioned in other studies.[16] They should be used as might otherwise be indicated for concomitant treatment of atrial fibrillation, coronary artery disease with recent acute coronary syndromes, heart failure, or hypertension.

Surgical and Endovascular Treatment

Monitoring with ultrasound or CT is recommended every 6-12 months for infrarenal or juxtarenal AAAs 4.0-5.4 cm in size and every 2-3 years for those that are <4.0 cm in size.[17] Aneurysm diameter is the strongest predictor of rupture; the risk of rupture does not exceed the risk of repair until the aneurysm expands to 5.5 cm. At a dimension of ≥5.5 cm, the risk of rupture increases markedly (*Table 6*). It is uncommon for AAA <5 cm to rupture.

In the United Kingdom Small Aneurysm trial, the risk of death due to rupture of AAAs between 4.0-5.5 cm in size over the 12 years of follow-up with clinical and ultrasound surveillance was lower than the risk of death from open AAA repair.[18] Among the participants who suffered a ruptured AAA, 25% died before reaching a hospital and another 50% died at the hospital prior to aortic repair. Overall 30-day survival after rupture was just 11%.[19]

The ADAM (Aneurysm Detection and Management) trial in patients ages 50-79 years (mostly men, most with a history of smoking) with a AAA diameter of 4.0-5.4 cm showed that mortality was similar in the patients randomized to immediate, elective surgical repair or ultrasound surveillance.[20] The relative risk for the primary endpoint of death from any case was 1.21 (95% confidence interval, 0.95-1.54). The total operative mortality was 2.7% in the immediate surgery group, and the AAA-related mortality was similar in both groups (3.0% with surgery and 2.6% with surveillance).

Diameter (cm)	Annual Risk of Rupture
<4.0	<0.5%
4.0 – 4.9	0.5 – 5.0%
5.0 – 5.9	3.0 – 15.0%
6.0 – 6.9	10.0 – 20.0%
7.0 – 7.9	20.0 – 40.0%
≥8.0	30.0 – 50.0%

Table 6
Annual Risk of Abdominal Aortic Rupture Based on Aneurysm Size

Symptomatic Patient	Any size
Asymptomatic Patient	≥5.5 cm* ≥1 cm per year growth

Table 7
Criteria for Surgical Intervention of AAAs by Size and Change in Size of Aneurysm

* Consider smaller (5.0 cm) diameter in women.

Based on these studies, the threshold for surgical intervention is an aneurysm dimension of ≥5.5 cm or a growth rate that exceeds 1.0 cm over a 12-month period. In good surgical candidates and women, many experts lower the threshold to 5.0 cm. Criteria for intervention in relation to AAA size and change in size are listed in *Table 7*.

Open surgical repair requires opening the aneurysm and placing an interposition graft. If the aneurysm extends distally beyond the aortic bifurcation, the repair may be carried into the common iliac arteries with a two-limb branched graft.

Alternatively, AAAs often can be repaired using EVAR techniques, with placement of a covered stent graft to bridge the aneurysm sac and exclude it from the circulation. The stent may be a straight tube graft or bifurcated, with branches extending into the common iliac arteries. Access is via the femoral artery.

When attempted, stent grafts are successfully deployed 98% of the time. However, one limitation of EVAR is that only about one-half of patients with AAAs have anatomy suitable for the procedure. A second limitation of the procedures is the occurrence of endoleaks. Per definition, an endoleak represents any persistent or new blood flow into the excluded aneurysm sac. A comprehensive classification and illustration of the types of endoleaks is presented in *Figure 5*.

Endoleaks may occur because of failure to adequately seal the proximal or distal end of the stent graft (type I endoleak), or because of retrograde flow from small branch arteries (such as lumbar arteries) back into the aneurysm sac (type II endoleak), a more common occurrence. Often, additional percutaneous procedures may be needed to treat endoleaks. Left untreated, they may lead to continued aortic expansion and rupture. Therefore, all patients with EVAR require routine monitoring by means of surveillance imaging. MRA has been shown to be effective in identifying endoleaks.

Multiple prospective, randomized, controlled trials comparing EVAR to open repair have shown significantly lower early mortality with EVAR. The DREAM (Dutch Randomized Endovascular Aneurysm Management) trial randomly assigned 351 patients to open repair or EVAR.[21] The EVAR 1 (Endovascular Aneurysm Repair Versus Open Repair in Patients with AAA) trial randomly assigned 1252 patients.[22] Although these trials showed that short-term (30-day) morbidity and mortality were significantly lower with EVAR, no significant differences in long-term outcomes were found.

A pooled analysis of these trials identified a 69% reduction in the risk of perioperative mortality for endovascular compared with open repair (Odds Ratio, 33; 95% CI, 0.17-0.64).[23] EVAR appears to be associated with a higher risk of future aortic rupture and the need for more secondary procedures.

Key Points

- Prospective trials have demonstrated that screening at-risk populations for AAAs is cost effective for aneurysm-related endpoints, and the US Preventive Services Task Force supports one-time screening by ultrasonography for AAA among men 65 to 75 years old who are current or former smokers.

- Medical therapy for AAA disease includes statins and aspirin for secondary prevention, smoking cessation, and blood pressure control.

- Elective repair of asymptomatic AAAs is recommended at a diameter of ≥5.5 cm, although in women, many experts lower the threshold to 5.0 cm because of their tendency to rupture at smaller diameters.

- Prospective randomized trials have shown significantly lower early mortality among patients treated with EVAR compared with open surgical repair; trials have not found significant differences in long-term survival.

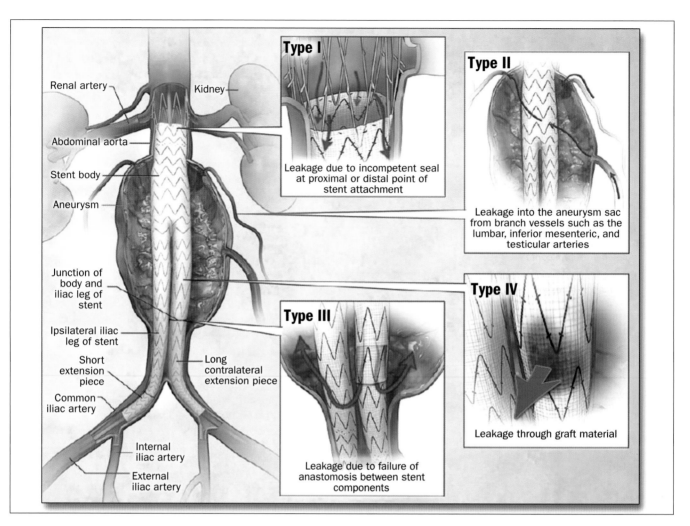

Figure 5

Classification of Endoleaks

The four types of leakage of blood into the aneurysm, or endoleak. Red arrows indicate blood flow.

Reproduced with permission from Greenhalgh RM, Powell JT. Endovascular repair of abdominal aortic aneurysm. N Eng J Med 2008;358:494-501.

References

1. He R, Guo DC, Estrera AL, et al. Characterization of the inflammatory and apoptotic cells in the aortas of patients with ascending thoracic aortic aneurysms and dissections. J Thorac Cardiovasc Surg 2006;131:671-8.

2. Tang PC, Coady MA, Lovoulos C, et al. Hyperplastic cellular remodeling of the media in ascending thoracic aortic aneurysms. Circulation 2005;112:1098-105.

3. Pannu H, Fadulu VT, Chang J, et al. Mutations in transforming growth factor-beta receptor type II cause familial thoracic aortic aneurysms and dissections. Circulation 2005;112:513-20.

4. Guo DC, Pannu H, Tran-Fadulu V, et al. Mutations in smooth muscle alpha-actin (ACTA2) lead to thoracic aortic aneurysms and dissections. Nat Genet 2007;39:1488-93.

5. Habashi JP, Judge DP, Holm TM, et al. Losartan, an AT1 antagonist, prevents aortic aneurysm in a mouse model of Marfan syndrome. Science 2006;312:117-21.

6. Lacro RV, Dietz HC, Sleeper LA, et al., on behalf of the Pediatric Heart Network Investigators. Atenolol versus losartan in children and young adults with Marfan's syndrome. N Engl J Med 2014;371:2061-71.

7. Hiratzka LF, Bakris GL, Beckman JA, et al. 2010 ACCF/AHA/ AATS/ACR/ASA/SCA/SCAI/SIR/STS/SVM guidelines for the diagnosis and management of patients with thoracic aortic disease. A report of the American College of Cardiology Foundation/American Heart Association Task Force on Practice Guidelines, American Association for Thoracic Surgery, American College of Radiology, American Stroke Association, Society of Cardiovascular Anesthesiologists, Society for Cardiovascular Angiography and Interventions, Society of Interventional Radiology, Society of Thoracic Surgeons, and Society for Vascular Medicine. J Am Coll Cardiol 2010;55:e27-e129.

8. Hiratzka LF, Creager MA, Isselbacher EM, et al. Surgery for aortic dilatation in patients with bicuspid aortic valves: a statement of clarification from the American College of Cardiology/American Heart Association Task Force on Clinical Practice Guidelines. J Am Coll Cardiol 2016;67:724-31.

9. Makaroun MS, Dillavou ED, Kee ST, et al. Endovascular treatment of thoracic aortic aneurysms: results of the phase II multicenter trial of the GORE TAG thoracic endoprosthesis. J Vasc Surg 2005;41:1-9.

10. Makaroun MS, Dillavou ED, Wheatley GH, Cambria RP, on behalf of the Gore TAG Investigators. Five-year results of endovascular treatment with the Gore TAG device compared with open repair of thoracic aortic aneurysms. J Vasc Surg 2008;47:912-8.

11. Biasetti J, Hussain F, Gasser TC. Blood flow and coherent vortices in the normal and aneurysmatic aortas: a fluid dynamical approach to intra-luminal thrombus formation. J R Soc Interface 2011;8:1449-61.

12. Abdul-Hussien H, Hanemaaijer R, Verheijen JH, van Bockel JH, Geelkerken RH, Lindeman JH. Doxycycline therapy for abdominal aneurysm: improved proteolytic balance through reduced neutrophil content. J Vasc Surg 2009;49:741-9.

13. Steinmetz EF, Buckley C, Shames ML, et al. Treatment with simvastatin suppresses the development of experimental abdominal aortic aneurysms in normal and hypercholesterolemic mice. Ann Surg 2005;241:92-101.

14. Wilson WR, Evans J, Bell PR, Thompson MM. HMG-CoA reductase inhibitors (statins) decrease MMP-3 and MMP-9 concentrations in abdominal aortic aneurysms. Eur J Vasc Endovasc Surg 2005;30: 259-62.

15. LeFevre ML, on behalf of the U.S. Preventive Services Task Force. Screening for abdominal aortic aneurysm: U.S. Preventive Services Task Force recommendation statement. Ann Intern Med 2014;161:281-90.

16. Gadowski GR, Pilcher DB, Ricci MA. Abdominal aortic aneurysm expansion rate: effect of size and beta-adrenergic blockade. J Vasc Surg 1994;19:727-31.

17. Anderson JL, Halperin JL, Albert N, et al. Management of patients with peripheral artery disease (compilation of 2005 and 2011 ACCF/AHA guideline recommendations): a report of the American College of Cardiology Foundation/American Heart Association Task Force on Practice Guidelines. J Am Coll Cardiol 2013;61:1555-70.

18. [No authors listed]. Mortality results for randomised controlled trial of early elective surgery or ultrasonographic surveillance for small abdominal aortic aneurysms. The UK Small Aneurysm Trial Participants. Lancet 1998;352:1649-55.

19. Brown LC, Powell JT. Risk factors for aneurysm rupture in patients kept under ultrasound surveillance. UK Small Aneurysm Trial Participants. Ann Surg 1999;230:289-96.

20. Lederle FA, Wilson SE, Johnson GR, et al., on behalf of the Aneurysm Detection and Management Veterans Affairs Cooperative Study Group. Immediate repair compared with surveillance of small abdominal aortic aneurysms. N Engl J Med 2002;346:1437-44.

21. Blankensteijn JD, de Jong SE, Prinssen M, et al., on behalf of the Dutch Randomized Endovascular Aneurysm Management (DREAM) Trial Group. Two-year outcomes after conventional or endovascular repair of abdominal aortic aneurysms. N Engl J Med 2005;352:2398-405.

22. United Kingdom EVAR Trial Investigators, Greenhalgh RM, Brown LC, Powell JT, et al. Endovascular versus open repair of abdominal aortic aneurysm. N Engl J Med 2010;362:1863-71.

23. Karthikesalingam A, Thompson MM. Vascular disease: repair of infrarenal aortic aneurysm--the debate is OVER. Nat Rev Cardiol 2013;10:122-4.

Acute Aortic Syndromes

Introduction

Acute aortic syndromes (AAS) comprise disease entities that threaten central aortic pressure, vital organ perfusion, survival, and functional recovery. They include aortic dissection, intramural hematoma (IMH), penetrating aortic ulcer (PAU), rapid aneurysm expansion, and trauma-induced aortic rupture.[1] Recent advances in genetic analysis, epidemiological understanding, and clinical care provide a greater range of tools with which to identify at-risk patients and diagnose AAS earlier in their natural history. Prompt delivery of appropriate medical, endovascular, and surgical therapy is a critical determinate of outcome.

Classification

AAS are defined according to the mechanism underlying aortic wall injury (*Table 1*). AAD is most commonly described according to the DeBakey[2] or Stanford[3] classification schemes (*Figure 1*). In the DeBakey system, a type I dissection originates within the ascending aorta and extends beyond the origin of the innominate artery. This is in contrast to a type II dissection that is confined to the ascending aorta or a type III dissection that begins distal to the origin of the left subclavian artery. The Stanford classification system, which will be referenced in the remainder of this module, divides dissections into two types: those that involve the ascending aorta constitute a type A dissection, whereas dissections that do not involve the ascending aorta are classified as type B dissections. In either schema, dissections originating in the transverse arch and extending distally are not strictly defined, but are most often aggregated with the most affected portion of contiguous aorta.

Bradley A. Maron, MD
This author has nothing to disclose.

Marc P. Bonaca, MD, MPH
Consultant Fees/Honoraria: AstraZeneca, Bayer, Merck, Roche; Research/Research Grants: Accumetrics, AstraZeneca, Beckman Coulter, Daiichi Sankyo, Eli Lilly, GlaxoSmithKline, Johnson & Johnson, Merck, Nanosphere, Ortho Clinical Diagnostics, Roche Diagnostics, Siemens Healthcare, Singulex.

Learner Objectives

Upon completion of this module, the reader will be able to:
1. Define each of the acute aortic syndromes (AAS).
2. Identify risk factors associated with the development of acute aortic dissection (AAD) and aortic rupture.
3. Recognize strengths and limitations of contemporary imaging modalities for diagnosis of AAS.
4. Recommend appropriate medical, endovascular, or surgical treatment for patients with AAS.
5. Recommend appropriate posthospital discharge care for AAS patients.

Key Point

- AAS include a spectrum of disease entities that threaten central aortic pressure, vital organ perfusion, survival, and functional recovery. These include aortic dissection, IMH, PAU, rapid aneurysm expansion, and trauma-induced aortic rupture. Aortic dissection is most commonly described according to the DeBakey[2] (I, II, III) or Stanford[3] (Type A, Type B) classification schemes.

Epidemiology

Declining autopsy rates, misdiagnosis, and an unknown contribution of AAS to prehospital sudden death are factors that obscure the true incidence of these events.[1,4] Data derived from large international registries estimate that the incidence of aortic aneurysm and dissection in the general population is 16.3 and 9.1 per 100,000 men and women, respectively, with a mean age of 63 years.[5-7] Importantly, disease rates vary (greatly) in accordance to the sample population. For example, patients with Marfan syndrome (MFS), which afflicts 1 in 5,000 individuals, are significantly more likely to develop an aortic dissection compared with the general population (discussed in the following section on Predisposing Risk Factors). IMH is believed to

Acute Aortic Syndrome	Definition
Aortic Dissection	The process by which a tear in the intima of the aorta allows access of blood into the media under systolic pressure, separation of the inner and outer media, and formation of true and false lumens.
Intramural Hematoma	A collection of blood within the wall of the aorta without a discernible entry tear.
Penetrating Aortic Ulcer	A crater-like outpouching of the aortic wall, originating most often as the growth of inflamed atherosclerotic plaque beyond the internal elastic lamina.
Rapid Aneurysm Expansion	Accelerated dilation of the aorta that is associated with weakening of the vessel wall and impending rupture.
Aortic Rupture	A tear (transection) through the entire wall of the aorta causing hemorrhage into the extravascular space.

Table 1
Acute Aortic Syndromes

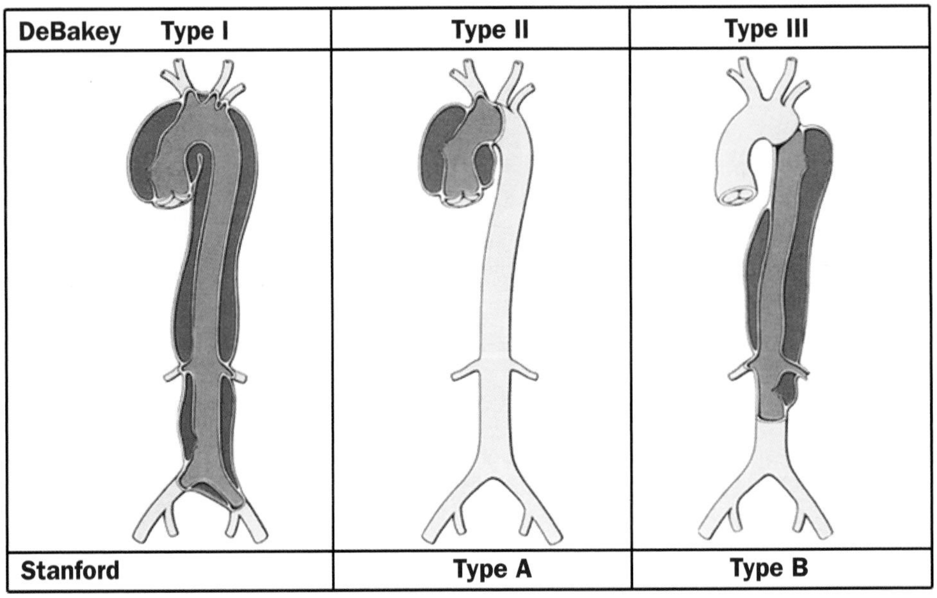

DeBakey		
Type I	Originates in the ascending aorta, propogates at least to the aortic arch and often beyond it distally
Type II	Originates in and is confined to the ascending aorta
Type III	Originates in the descending aorta and extends distally down the aorta or, rarely, retrograde into the aortic arch and ascending aorta

Stanford	
Type A	All dissections involving the ascending aorta, regardless of the site of origin
Type B	All dissections not involving the ascending aorta

Acute: Presentation ≤2 weeks following symptom onset
Chronic: Presentation >2 weeks following symptom onset

Figure 1
Aortic Dissection Type According to the DeBakey and Stanford Classification Systems

Modified from Nienaber CA, Eagle KA. Aortic dissection: new frontiers in diagnosis and management: part I: from etiology to diagnostic strategies. Circulation 2003;108:628-35.

Genetic Factors	Comments
Marfan Syndrome (MFS)	FBN-1 mutation Fibrillin deficiency
Ehlers-Danlos Syndrome	COL3A1 mutation ~50% are sporadic
Familial Thoracic Aortic Aneurysm Disease	MYH11 mutation ACTA2 mutation Others
Bicuspid Aortic Valve (BAV) Disease	Most common congenital heart defect Associated aortopathy with features similar to MFS
Loeys-Dietz Syndrome	TGFBR1 and TGFBR2 mutations
Aortic Coarctation	Uncommonly diagnosed in adulthood May be part of BAV disease
Noonan Syndrome	PTPN11 mutation (most common)
Turner Syndrome	XO karyotype
Polycystic Kidney Disease	PKD1 and PDK2 mutations

Table 2a

Genetic Risk Factors for Acute Aortic Syndromes

Acquired Factors	Comments
Hypertension	Present in ~65% of cases

Iatrogenic	Most commonly a complication of:
	    cardiac surgery
	    cardiac catheterization

Pregnancy	Generally uncommon 50% of all dissection in women <40 years of age are peripartum
Inflammatory Aortitis	Takayasu's disease Giant cell aortitis Behcet's disease Relapsing polychondritis Systemic lupus erythematosus *Not* in syphilis-induced aortitis
Cocaine Amphetamines	↑ Wall stress, tachycardia, catecholamine-induced shear stress ↑ Endothelial dysfunction

Table 2b

Acquired Risk Factors for Acute Aortic Syndromes

account for up to 13% of AAS.[5,6] Aortic rupture may occur as a complication of type A dissection, but is rare outside the setting of trauma. By some estimates, aortic rupture accounts for 20% of motor vehicle collision-related fatalities.

Predisposing Risk Factors

The likelihood of developing an AAS is influenced by genetic and acquired risk factors that weaken the medial layer of the aortic wall (*Table 2a, b*). Cystic medial degeneration describes the noninflammatory loss of elastic fibers in the aortic media due to the accumulation of mucopolysaccharides and vascular smooth muscle cell degeneration. In many cases, however, pockets (cysts) of mucopolysaccharide accumulation may not be evident on pathologic review, and hence, medial degeneration may be a more universal term. The functional consequences of these changes include weakening of the aortic wall with a loss of tensile strength. Importantly, the aortopathy predisposing to AAD reflects a wide variety of etiologies; thus, the presence of medial degeneration is not pathognomonic for any single cause of aortic dissection.

Genetic Risk Factors
Marfan Syndrome
Numerous genetic etiologies have been implicated in the pathophysiology of AAS. MFS is the most common genetic cause of AAD and occurs owing to mutations in the gene encoding for fibrillin-1 (*FBN1*), which is a major component of microfibrils that form a structure-supporting sheath around elastin. Dysfunctional microfibrils result in the loss of intercellular adhesions and ultimately in a cardiovascular syndrome that includes aneurysms of the aorta (most often affecting the root and sinuses of Valsalva), dilation of the proximal main pulmonary artery, myxomatous thickening of the atrioventricular valves, mitral valve prolapse, and mitral annular calcification.[8] In addition, structurally

Negative MFS Family History	Positive MFS Family History	Systemic Score (points)
Aorta z score >2 and: Ectopic lentis *or* FBN-1 mutation *or* Systemic score >7	Ectopic lentis *or* Systemic score >7 *or* Aortic z score ≥2 above 20 years of age *or* Aortic z score ≥3 below 20 years of age	Wrist/thumb sign: 3 Pectus carinatum: 2 Hindfoot deformity: 2 Pneumothorax: 2 Dural ectasia: 2 Protrusio acetabuli: 2 Decreased upper segment/lower segment ratio: 1 Scoliosis: 1 Reduced elbow extension: 1 Facial features: 1 Skin striae: 1 Myopia: 1 Mitral valve prolapse: 1

Table 3

Selected Criteria for the Diagnosis of Marfan Syndrome

MFS = Marfan syndrome.

Adapted from Loeys BL, Dietz HC, Braverman AC, et al. The revised Ghent nosology for the Marfan syndrome. J Med Genet 2010;47:476-85.

abnormal fibrillin is associated with diminished binding of fibrillin by transforming growth factor-beta (TGF-β) and subsequently increased accumulation of TGF-β. Overactivation of TGF-β signaling in the aorta, in turn, has emerged as a contemporary treatment target in MFS. Angiotensin-receptor blocker therapy decreases the rate of aorta dilation in this disease with efficacy akin to therapy with beta-adrenergic receptor antagonists.[9,10]

The diagnosis of MFS is established primarily on clinical grounds. In the setting of a family history of MFS, the presence of ectopia lentis or aortic dilatation (z score ≥2 for those >20 years of age) is sufficient to secure the diagnosis.[11] Because up to one-third of cases present in patients without an affected parent,[8] strategies to diagnose MFS exist that rely on clinical examination findings, imaging, and molecular testing (*Table 3*). Furthermore, MFS variants that affect primarily the cardiovascular system (i.e., formes frustes) have been described and are important to recognize clinically due to their association with aortic aneurysm and dissection. These include the MASS phenotype (myopia, mitral valve prolapse, nonprogressive aortic root dilation, skeletal abnormalities, and striae) and familial thoracic aortic aneurysm disease. Familial thoracic aortic aneurysm disease also has been mapped to mutations in *MYH11* and *ACTA2*.[12,13]

Ehlers-Danlos Syndrome
Vascular Ehlers-Danlos syndrome (i.e., type IV) is a rare autosomal dominant disorder that occurs due to a mutation in the *COL3A1* gene encoding for type III procollagen synthesis. Notably, up to one-half of cases are not inherited and are believed to be sporadic.[14] Vascular Ehlers-Danlos syndrome is associated with an increased risk of spontaneous vascular or visceral rupture, with vascular complications tending to involve the iliac, splenic, or renal arteries, as well as the aorta. In vascular Ehlers-Danlos syndrome, aortic aneurysm, dissection, and rupture

have been reported, and mortality rates are elevated significantly compared with the normal population, with cumulative survival of approximately 50% at age 40 years.[15]

Loeys-Dietz Syndrome
Autosomal dominant mutations to the *TGFBR1* and *TGFBR2* genes result in overactive TGF-β signal transduction that destabilizes connective tissue and causes a constellation of findings that characterize Loeys-Dietz syndrome, including craniofacial abnormalities (e.g., hypertelorism, cleft palate, others), as well as tortuosity, aneurysm, and increased predilection to dissection of the aorta and branch vessels.[16] In contrast to other aortopathies, Loeys-Dietz syndrome is associated with rupture at near normal vessel dimensions that may occur early in life, with vascular catastrophes reported in patients as young as 6 months of age.[17] Therefore, yearly echocardiography, strict management of blood pressure (BP), avoidance of contact or competitive athletics, and early surgical referral are recommended for Loeys-Dietz syndrome patients.[18]

Bicuspid Aortic Valve Disease and Other Genetic Risk Factors
Bicuspid aortic valve disease is the most common congenital heart defect, affecting 1-2% of the general population, and is present in a male-to-female ratio of 3:1.[19] Compared with the general population, affected individuals demonstrate a relative risk for aortic dissection and aortic aneurysm of 8.5 and 86.2, respectively.[20] Although the mechanism by which to account for the aortopathy of bicuspid aortic valve is unresolved, disrupted laminar flow within the postvalvular segment of the proximal aorta is associated with medial degeneration, smooth muscle cell disarray, and fragmentation of elastin.[19] Other genetic syndromes associated with an increased rate of aortic aneurysm/dissection include aortic coarctation, Noonan's syndrome, Turner's syndrome, and polycystic kidney disease.

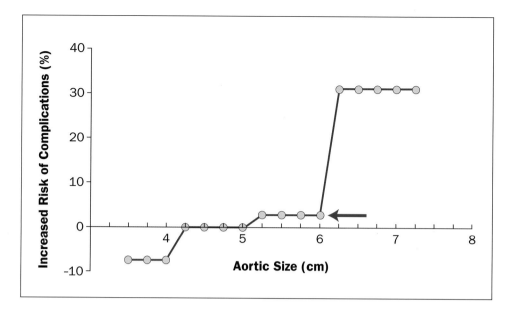

Figure 2

Influence of Aortic Size on Cumulative Lifetime Incidence of Natural Complications of Aortic Aneurysm

An inflection point in the risk of aneurysm complications (i.e., dissection, rupture) is observed in non-Marfan syndrome patients at an aortic diameter >6 cm (blue arrow).

Reproduced with permission from Elefteriades JA. Natural history of thoracic aortic aneurysm: indications for surgery, and surgical versus nonsurgical risks. Ann Thorac Surg 2002;74:S1877-80.

Acquired Risk Factors

Systemic hypertension and tobacco use are the most common acquired (i.e., modifiable) risk factors for aortic dissection. Recreational use of cocaine and methamphetamine are recognized increasingly as stimulators of aortic vascular injury. Other acquired risk factors for aortic dissection include inflammatory diseases of the large arteries, such as Takayasu's disease, giant cell aortitis, Behçet's disease, relapsing polychondritis, systemic lupus erythematosus, and rarely, inflammatory bowel disease-associated vasculitis.[21] However, vasculopathies characterized by significant replacement fibrosis and subsequent scarring of the blood vessel wall, as occurs in response to *Treponema pallidum* infection (i.e., syphilis), are generally associated with aortopathy and aneurysm and not with an increased risk for aortic dissection.

Changes in circulating blood volume, increased levels of the vascular effectors relaxin and estrogen, Valsalva maneuver-mediated increases in intrathoracic pressure during labor, and undiagnosed MFS or other connective tissue diseases are predisposing factors for aortic dissection during pregnancy. While aortic dissection occurs most commonly during the third trimester of pregnancy, event risk also is increased in the early postpartum phase. Although these events are rare and most commonly occur in the context of a previously unrecognized connective tissue abnormality, up to 50% of all dissections in women <40 years of age occur in the peripartum period.[22]

Iatrogenic causes of aortic dissection account for up to 5% of all events and occur most commonly during cardiac surgery or catheterization. Peripheral vascular disease, tobacco use, and a history of systemic hypertension are associated with increased risk of iatrogenic dissection.[22] In one series of patients undergoing aortic surgery, the rate of unintended aortic injury, including dissection, was approximately 0.2%, which was attributed to evidence of medial degeneration on postprocedural histological analysis.[23] This finding raises speculation that patients affected by iatrogenic aortic injury may be at elevated risk due to an abnormal vascular substrate.[24]

Key Points

- Mutations in the *FBN1*, *TGFB1/2*, and *COL3A* genes cause Marfan, Loeys-Dietz, and vascular Ehlers-Danlos syndromes, respectively, which are three genetic risk factors for aortic aneurysm and dissection.

- Acquired risk factors for aortic dissection include systemic hypertension, tobacco use, and the development of various autoimmune diseases. Aortic rupture (transection) most commonly occurs following deceleration injuries (e.g., motor vehicle collision).

Pathophysiology

Aortic Dissection

There is a positive sigmoid relationship between thoracic aortic diameter and probability of aortic dissection/rupture with a steep upward inflection point at 6 cm (*Figure 2*).[25] Nevertheless, dissection often will occur at much smaller aortic diameters.[26]

In 80-90% of cases of acute syndromes, an intimal tear is identified at autopsy or through advanced imaging of the aorta and is most likely to occur at points of high shear or mechanical stress, such as within a few centimeters of the aortic valve for type A dissections and just distal to the insertion of the ligamentum arteriosum for type B dissections.[21] Propagation of the dissecting hematoma may occur anterograde or retrograde, resulting in involvement of both the ascending and descending aorta. Re-entry sites may be multiple.

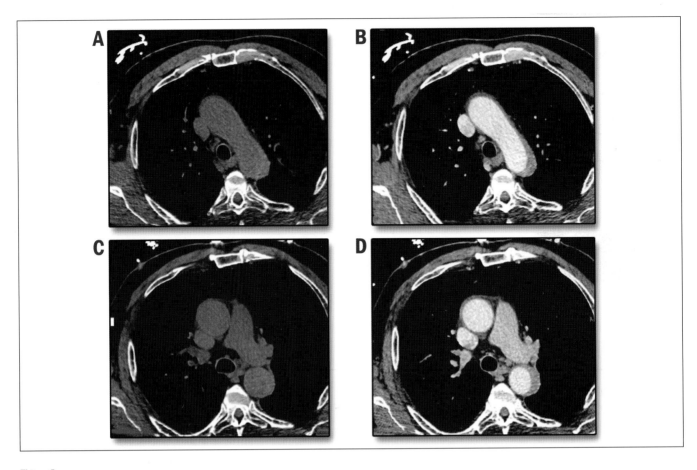

Figure 3

Aortic Intramural Hematoma Seen on Computed Tomography Imaging

Noncontrast (**panels A, C**) and contrast (**panels B, D**) computed tomography demonstrating an intramural hematoma originating in the distal ascending aorta and arch (**panels A, B**) and extending into the descending aorta (**panels C, D**).

Reproduced with permission from Bonaca MP, O'Gara PT. Diagnosis and management of acute aortic syndromes: dissection, intramural hematoma, and penetrating aortic ulcer. Curr Cardiol Rep. 2014;16:536.

The patency of the false lumen of a dissection influences the natural history of the disease. Generally, either complete thrombosis or patent entry and re-entry tears are associated with favorable outcomes, while partial thrombosis of the false lumen is associated with increased false lumen pressures and predicts future dissection-associated complications, possibly due to increased compression of the true lumen by the false lumen or owing to sustained inflammation-mediated injury to the aortic wall. Tsai et al. showed that partial false lumen thrombosis was associated with reduced long-term survival among patients with type B aortic dissection and proposed that hemodynamic forces within the false lumen lead ultimately to progressive aneurysm formation or rupture.[27] Patency of the false lumen is common among patients with MFS and aortic dissection and could be a risk factor for late complications.

Clinical manifestations of aortic dissection are intimately related to the site of entry, course of the propagating hematoma, and branch vessel compromise. The dissection plane of a type A dissection may propagate retrograde across the origin of the coronary arteries, particularly the right coronary artery, causing myocardial ischemia, or involve the aortic annulus, with resultant valvular regurgitation. Rupture into the pericardial space can result in tamponade and early death. End-organ malperfusion syndromes due to aortic branch vessel compromise equate with increased morbidity and mortality.[21]

Aortic Intramural Hematoma

IMH is defined as a collection of blood within the media of the aorta in the absence of dissection flap or a detectable entry tear (*Figure 3*).[21] It is believed to occur as a result of spontaneous bleeding within the wall of the aorta from damaged vasa vasorum. The probability of IMH evolving into an acute aortic event is not fully characterized, although in one report from the International Registry of Acute Aortic Dissection of 178 patients, the incidence of IMH among AAS patients was as high as 25%, with the descending aorta most often affected.[28] Data from other series have reported that IMH is a strong risk factor for the development of aortic aneurysm, with coincidence rates of 50-60%.[29]

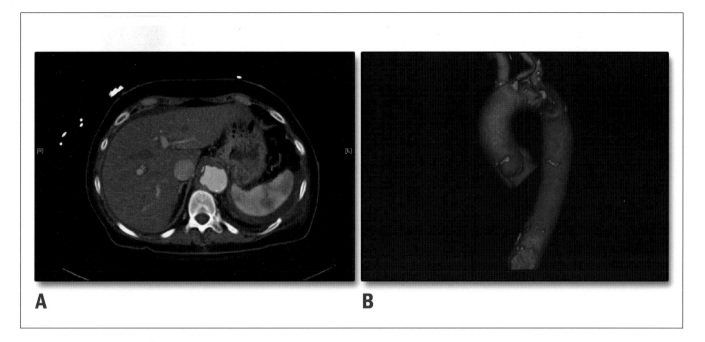

Figure 4

Penetrating Atherosclerotic Ulcer Seen on Computed Tomography Imaging

Two-dimensional (**panel A**) and three-dimensional (**panel B**) reconstruction computed tomography angiography from a patient with multiple penetrating aortic ulcers.

Reproduced with permission from Bonaca MP, O'Gara PT. Diagnosis and management of acute aortic syndromes: dissection, intramural hematoma, and penetrating aortic ulcer. Curr Cardiol Rep. 2014;16:536.

Diagnosis of IMH is most often accomplished using transesophageal echocardiography (TEE), computed tomography angiography (CTA), or magnetic resonance angiography (MRA), with demonstration of partial or circumferential wall thickening or the presence of a fresh hematoma in the vessel wall (crescentic appearance). CTA outperforms TEE as a diagnostic imaging modality; however, the initial noncontrast image sequence is most sensitive for identifying isolated IMH. The natural history of IMH is variable: spontaneous resorption may occur in up to a third of cases, although if present in the ascending aorta, a diameter of >11 mm is predictive of complications, including death, and the need for surgical repair.[21,30,31] The incidence rates of aortic regurgitation and pulse deficits are lower with IMH compared with dissection. Over time, approximately 10% of patients with IMH will evolve a classic dissection, and 50-60% will develop true or false aortic aneurysms.

Penetrating Atherosclerotic Aortic Ulcer

The perturbation of stable aortic atherosclerotic plaques from inflammation or shear stress may result in subsequent erosion across the internal elastic membrane into and beyond the media of the aorta (*Figure 4*). PAU depth >1.0 cm, diameter >2.0 cm, and location in the proximal aspect of the descending aorta is associated with worse outcomes. Ulceration may lead to false aneurysm development, rupture, or medial propagation. For uncomplicated lesions not associated with an enlarging false aneurysm, IMH,

or dissection, serial imaging and a conservative medical strategy are recommended (discussed later in the section on *Management of Aortic Dissection*).

Clinical Presentation

History

A high clinical index of suspicion for aortic dissection in appropriate patients is necessary to avoid misdiagnosis, as an increase in mortality rate of 0.22% per hour is observed during the first 24 hours in type A dissection patients, which is increased to 0.77% per hour for such patients managed medically.[32]

Point-of-care clinical prediction rules recently have been validated to provide a simple and uniform strategy for determining the likelihood of dissection at the patient's bedside (*Table 4*).[33]

Chest pain is the most common presenting symptom among patients with AAD (*Table 5*). The quality of chest pain tends to be described by patients as severe at onset, ripping, or tearing. Radiation of discomfort anteriorly is suggestive of type A aortic dissection, while radiation of discomfort to the lower back or abdominal region is suggestive of type B dissection. Syncope is a particularly concerning symptom of aortic dissection and should raise immediate concern for cerebral malperfusion or cardiac tamponade. Other major symptoms associated with worse

High-Risk Conditions 28.1%	High-Risk Pain Features 87.5%	High-Risk Exam Features 51.0%
• Marfan Syndrome • Family history of aortic disease • Known aortic valve disease • Recent aortic manipulation • Known thoracic aortic aneurysm	**Chest, back, or abdominal pain described as:** · Abrupt in onset · Severe in intensity · Ripping or tearing	**Evidence of perfusion deficit** (pulse deficit, systolic blood pressure differential, focal neurologic deficit in conjunction with pain) **Murmur of aortic insufficiency** (new or not known to be old and in conjunction with pain) **Hypotension or shock state**

Table 4

The Percentage of Patients in the International Registry of Acute Aortic Dissection (IRAD) (1996-2009) With Each Category of Risk Marker Present on Presentation

The aortic dissection detection (ADD) score aims to enhance early diagnosis of acute aortic dissection.

The ADD score is calculated by determining the number of categories in which a feature is present in patients with symptoms suggestive of acute aortic dissection. For example, in a patient with a family history of aortic disease (high-risk condition) and the abrupt onset of chest pain (high-risk pain feature), the ADD score would be 2. Likewise, the ADD score is 2 in a patient with Marfan syndrome (high-risk condition) and a blood pressure differential (high-risk exam feature).

The ADD scale may therefore provide the clinician with a simple and effective bedside method to inform further diagnostic testing and/or treatment in patients with suspected aortic dissection. In the IRAD evaluation, only 4.3% had an ADD score of 0, 36.5% had an ADD score of 1, and 59.2% had an ADD score of 2 or 3. Importantly, the negative predictive value for acute aortic dissection in patients with an ADD score of 0 has not yet been established.

Reproduced with permission from Rogers AM, Hermann LK, Booher AM, et al. Sensitivity of the aortic dissection detection risk score, a novel guideline-based tool for identification of acute aortic dissection on initial presentation. Circulation 2011;123:2213-8.

Symptom	Mean Sensitivity % (Range)
Any pain	90 (85-94)
Chest Pain	67 (56-77)
Anterior Chest Pain	57 (48-66)
Posterior Chest Pain	32 (24-40)
Back Pain	32 (19-47)
Abdominal Pain	23 (16-31)
Sudden-Onset Pain	84 (80-89)
Severe Pain	90 (88-92)
Ripping/Tearing Pain	39 (14-69)
Migrating Pain	31 (12-55)
Syncope	9 (8-12)

Table 5

The Average Sensitivity of Various Clinical Features Reported in Patients With Acute Thoracic Aortic Dissection

Data are derived from a meta-analysis involving 16 different studies and 1,553 patients.

Adapted from Klompas M. Does this patient have an acute thoracic aortic dissection? JAMA 2002;287:2262-72.

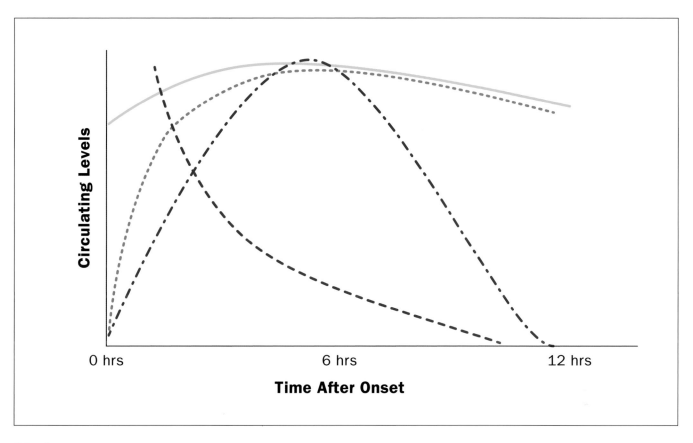

Figure 5
Circulating Level of Aortic Biomarkers After Acute Dissection

Reproduced with permission from Trimarchi S, Sangiorgi G, Sang X, et al. In search of blood tests for thoracic aortic diseases. Ann Thorac Surg 2010;90:1735-42.

outcome in aortic dissection include abdominal pain and paraplegia, which may occur in the presence of impaired blood flow to the spinal cord.

Physical Examination

Patients with AAD often present acutely ill. Hypertension may be observed in either type A or type B aortic dissection. If present, an aortic regurgitation murmur is often faint, short in duration, and low pitched. Identifying pulse deficits is critical, as this predicts mortality in AAD.[34] Patients also should be evaluated for clinical signs of cardiac tamponade such as pulsus paradoxus and elevation of the jugular venous pressure. Serosanguinous pleural effusions (left > right) are reported in acute type B aortic dissection and should be considered in patients for whom dullness to percussion or decreased breath sounds are observed on clinical examination.

Key Point

- Severe and abrupt onset chest pain is the most common symptom in AAD.

Biomarkers

A low D-dimer (<500 ng/ml) discovered at the time of presentation suggests against AAD and may be a useful screening tool to exclude the diagnosis in low-probability patients. An elevated D-dimer is a nonspecific finding and does not establish the diagnosis of aortic dissection. Elevated circulating levels of smooth muscle myosin heavy chain protein (>2.5 mcg/L) in the first few hours after onset of symptoms raise the clinical index of suspicion for acute type A aortic dissection. The role of these and other biomarkers, such as C-reactive protein and soluble elastin fragment for aortic dissection diagnosis or risk stratification, continues to evolve (*Figure 5*).

Diagnostic Imaging

The chest X-ray is abnormal in the majority of aortic dissection patients, but is generally nonspecific and alone is not sufficient for establishing an accurate diagnosis. Common findings include widening of the mediastinum and angulation of the aortic border. Similarly, the electrocardiogram is often abnormal but nondiagnostic. Importantly, although present in <4% of patients, the presence of new Q waves or ST-segment elevation may

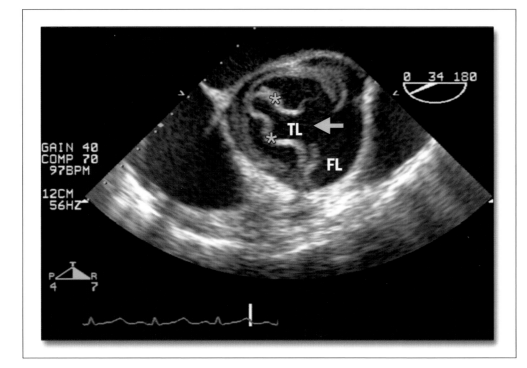

Figure 6

Transesophageal Echocardiographic Capture of Aortic Dissection

A type A aortic dissection visualized by transesophageal echocardiography demonstrates a communication (arrow) through the dissection flap between the true lumen (TL) and false lumen (FL).

*Aortic valve leaflets.

Reproduced with permission from Meredith EL, Masani ND. Echocardiography in the emergency assessment of acute aortic syndromes. Eur J Echocardiogr 2009;10:i31-9.

indicate coronary involvement with type A dissection and must be considered carefully to avoid inappropriate delivery of fibrinolytic/reperfusion therapy.

Transesophageal Echocardiography

TEE is an effective modality for diagnosing aortic dissection as well as several complications, such as pericardial effusion (*Figure 6*). When combined with transthoracic echocardiography, the sensitivity and specificity of these tests approach 99% and 89%, respectively.[35]

Identifying the false lumen from the true lumen may be difficult with B-mode imaging alone, and in cases for which the false lumen is large, this distinction should not be made according only to vessel diameter. Continuous wave Doppler interrogation may be used in these cases to measure the velocity time integral of blood flow within each lumen, thus providing an estimation of intraluminal pressure to distinguish between the true and false lumens. The distal ascending aorta, anterior aspect of the aortic arch, and regions of the aorta anterior to the cartilaginous trachea are often obstructed from view with TEE.

Computed Tomography Angiography

The diagnostic accuracy of 64-slice CTA approaches 100% for aortic dissection.[21,36] Contrast enhancement allows thorough anatomical characterization of the dissection plane, including detailed characterization of distal branch vessel involvement. Additional benefits of CTA include rapid image acquisition and the availability of emergency department scanners at most hospitals. Limitations of CTA include patient exposure to radiation and contrast. Test accuracy may be influenced adversely by motion artifact, and therefore, optimal protocols using electrocardiogram gating should be considered to maximize diagnostic

accuracy. In addition, protocols that assess left ventricular (LV) or aortic valve function may provide additional information. CTA has become the first imaging modality of choice for suspected AAD worldwide.

Magnetic Resonance Angiography

MRA offers excellent spatial resolution for geometric and volumetric analysis of aortic dissections and enhances sensitivity for detecting IMH and PAU. In most cases, weighted imaging protocols also allow for distinction between a thrombosed versus patent false lumen. In contrast to CTA, MRA provides information on LV and aortic valve function, as well as quantifying aortic regurgitation. MRA is often more useful in stable follow-up rather than in the acute diagnosis due to availability and the time required for image acquisition (*Figure 7*). The lack of ionizing radiation makes MRA an attractive modality for long-term surveillance.

Invasive Aortography

Limited diagnostic sensitivity and the availability of other more accurate but less invasive diagnostic tests have resulted in a substantial decline in the application of invasive aortography as a first-line test for the diagnosis of aortic dissection. This strategy remains an option in specific circumstances, such as to evaluate aortic dissection in patients misdirected to the cardiac catheterization lab for evaluation of presumed ischemic coronary disease. Under these clinical circumstances, intravascular ultrasound also may be utilized. The diagnostic accuracy of intravascular ultrasound is nearly 100% for aortic dissection, and is particularly useful for defining circumferential extent of disease as well as located dissection entry points.

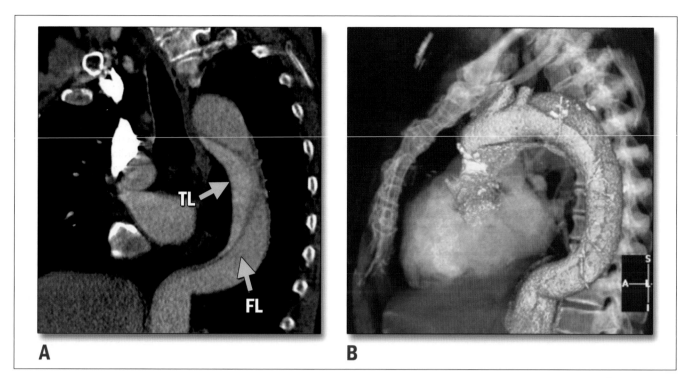

Figure 7

Computed Tomography Angiography and Three-Dimensional Reconstructed Images of Stanford Type A Dissection

Panel A: Coronal computed tomography angiography images delineate the intimal flap that separates the true lumen (TL) from the false lumen (FL).

Panel B: Three-dimensional reconstruction imaging in the same patient provides enhanced spatial resolution postsurgical repair of the aortic dissection and the surrounding anatomic structures.

Reproduced with permission from Maron BA, O'Gara PT. Pathophysiology, clinical evaluation, and medical management of aortic dissection. In: Creager M, Beckman JA, Loscalzo J, eds. Vascular Medicine: A Companion to Braunwald's Heart Disease. 2nd ed. Philadelphia: Saunders; 2013:687-96.

Coronary angiography is not routinely indicated in the management of patients with AAD. On the other hand, coronary angiography prior to elective repair of chronic stable type A dissections is reasonable, particularly for patients with a known history of ischemic heart disease.

> ### Key Point
>
> - TEE, CTA, and MRA are effective imaging modalities for diagnosis of AAD. CTA has become the most widely used initial test to diagnose suspected aortic dissection.

Management of Aortic Dissection

The management of aortic dissection proceeds methodically and expeditiously, often combining medical and surgical therapies. The clinical indications for the use of endovascular aortic stent grafts for type B dissection continue to evolve. One proposed pathway algorithm for the management of patients with AAD is provided in *Figure 8*.

Medical Therapy

Medical therapy with intravenous agents to control heart rate (HR) and BP is the cornerstone of the initial therapeutic strategy for all patients with a suspected AAS. Exceptions to this rule include unstable patients with cardiogenic shock and profound systemic hypotension, typically due to type A aortic dissection complicated by aortic rupture or cardiac tamponade. In these cases, volume resuscitation is indicated as a temporizing measure prior to emergent surgery without delay. Delay for procedures such as pericardiocentesis generally is not advised. Pericardiocentesis may have the added disadvantage of acutely destabilizing a vulnerable patient.

Short-acting beta-adrenergic receptor antagonists are preferred first-line agents, as these drugs reduce the rate of pressure development (i.e., change in pressure divided by change in time [dP/dT]) by decreasing both LV contractility and HR (*Table 6*).[37] The target HR in the acute phase of management is ~60 bpm. In patients requiring additional therapy to achieve a target BP of ~110 mm Hg, the intravenous administration of short-acting direct vasodilators is recommended, such as

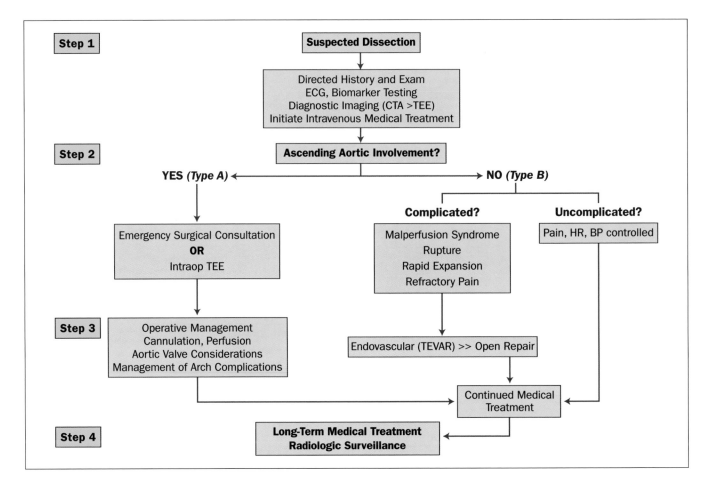

Figure 8
Proposed Management Pathway for Acute Aortic Dissection

In Step 1, a high index of clinical suspicion for acute aortic dissection should prompt early diagnostic testing while medical therapy is initiated. Step 2 involves the determination of ascending aortic involvement, which influences significantly the importance of emergency surgical consultation. In Step 3, patients with type A aortic dissection are referred for surgery and patients with complicated type B aortic dissection are referred for endovascular therapy or surgery. Patients with uncomplicated type B aortic dissection are continued on medical therapy and monitored for changes in clinical status. In Step 4, a care plan is established that emphasizes the importance of long-term medical therapy, radiologic surveillance, and lifestyle modifications to decrease the risk of postdissection complications. Long-term medical therapy should include beta-receptor antagonists and angiotensin-receptor blockers or angiotensin-converting enzyme inhibitors to achieve a resting HR of ≤60 bpm and BP of <130/80 mm Hg, respectively.

BP = blood pressure; CTA = computed tomography angiography; ECG = electrocardiogram; HR = heart rate; TEE = transesophageal echocardiography; TEVAR = thoracic endovascular aneurysm repair.

Legend modified from Maron BA, O'Gara PT. Pathophysiology, clinical evaluation, and medical management of aortic dissection. In: Creager M, Beckman JA, Loscalzo J, eds. Vascular Medicine: A Companion to Braunwald's Heart Disease. 2nd ed. Philadelphia: Saunders; 2013:687-96.

Image modified from Hiratzka LF, Bakris GL, Beckman JA, et al. 2010 ACCF/AHA/AATS/ACR/ASA/SCA/SCAI/SIR/STS/SVM guidelines for the diagnosis and management of patients with thoracic aortic disease. A report of the American College of Cardiology Foundation/American Heart Association Task Force on Practice Guidelines, American Association for Thoracic Surgery, American College of Radiology, American Stroke Association, Society of Cardiovascular Anesthesiologists, Society for Cardiovascular Angiography and Interventions, Society of Interventional Radiology, Society of Thoracic Surgeons, and Society for Vascular Medicine. J Am Coll Cardiol 2010;55:e27-129.

nitroprusside, labetalol, enalaprilat, hydralazine, or nicardipine.[38] Vasodilators should not be added prior to beta-blockade as this may increase HR and the rate of LV pressure rise (dP/dT). Other supportive measures may be necessary to alleviate hypoxemia, patient discomfort, and anxiety, which collectively may exacerbate dissection pathophysiology.

Surgery

The indications for surgical repair of acute and chronic aortic dissection are outlined in *Table 7*.

Emergency surgery is recommended for all patients with acute type A aortic dissection, as well as for patients with type A IMH, in the absence of extreme morbidity. The potential for

Therapy	Dose	Receptor Selectivity and Half-Life
Metoprolol	5 mg bolus every 5 minutes for 3 doses; additional doses of 5-10 mg every 4-6 hrs as needed.	$ß_1 > ß_2$ 3-6 hours.
Labetalol	10-20 mg bolus, repeat 20-40 mg bolus every 10-15 min as needed. Maintenance infusion 1-2 mg/min; maximum total dose of 300 mg.	$α_1$-, $ß_1$-, and $ß_2$ ~5.5 hours.
Esmolol	0.5 mg/kg bolus, then 50 mcg/kg/min infusion.	$ß_1$ 9 minutes.
Propranolol	0.05–0.15 mg/kg every 4-6 hrs as needed.	$ß_1 \approx ß_2$ 5-7 hours.

Table 6

Intravenous ß-adrenergic Receptor Antagonists for the Management of Acute Aortic Dissection

Reproduced with permission from Maron BA, O'Gara PT. Pathophysiology, clinical evaluation, and medical management of aortic dissection. In: Creager M, Beckman JA, Loscalzo J, eds. Vascular Medicine: A Companion to Braunwald's Heart Disease. 2nd ed. Philadelphia: Elsevier; 2016.

Acute Dissection	Chronic Dissection
Type A: All patients	**Type A:** Maximal dimension ≥5.5 cm Increase in dimension ≥1 cm/yr Severe aortic regurgitation Symptoms suggestive of expansion or compression
Type B: With Complications Rupture Extension Rapid Aneurysm Expansion Malperfusion Syndrome Marfan Syndrome?	**Type B:** Maximal dimension ≥6 cm Increase in dimension ≥1 cm/yr Symptoms suggestive of expansion or compression

Table 7

Indications for Surgery in Acute and Chronic Aortic Dissection

Adapted from Hiratzka LF, Bakris GL, Beckman JA, et al. 2010 ACCF/AHA/AATS/ ACR/ASA/SCA/SCAI/SIR/ STS/SVM guidelines for the diagnosis and management of patients with thoracic aortic disease. J Am Coll Cardiol 2010;55:e27-e129.

aortic arch reconstruction, coronary artery reimplantation, aortic valve repair or replacement, and branch vessel repair is dependent on aortic dissection anatomy and assessed on an individual basis. Surgical repair of chronic stable type A aortic dissection is recommended in the presence of significant aortic valve dysfunction (regurgitation), LV cavity dilation, or LV systolic dysfunction. Likewise, surgery to treat an ascending aortic aneurysm is indicated for a maximal dimension ≥5.5 cm or ≥4.5 cm in MFS patients or accelerated dilation at a rate of ≥1 cm/year.[1]

Surgery typically consists of resection and replacement of the dissected ascending aorta using an aortic root graft, although aortic valve resuspension or use of a composite Valsalva valve-graft conduit with reimplantation of the coronary arteries may be required, depending on the extent of root involvement and the mechanism of any associated aortic regurgitation. Techniques for managing complex arch dissections and branch vessel involvement with bifurcated, debranching grafts are beyond the scope of this module. Cannulation for cardiopulmonary bypass is usually performed via the right axillary artery, and a period

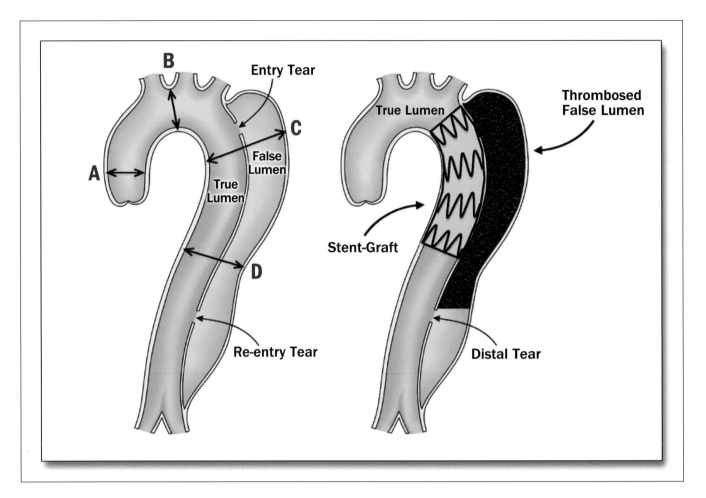

Figure 9

Endovascular Stent-Graft in Type B Dissection

Cartoon demonstrating the typical features of type B dissection with flow in both the true and the expanded false lumen, resulting from a proximal entry tear (left). A stent graft was placed to scaffold the dissected aorta and to seal the entry site, resulting in reconstruction of the true lumen with subsequent false-lumen thrombosis (right). Levels were defined as (**A**) at the sinotubular junction, (**B**) at the center of the arch between innominate artery and left common carotid artery, (**C**) at the level of the maximum aortic diameter, and (**D**) at the diaphragmatic hiatus.

Reproduced with permission from Nienaber CA, Rousseau H, Eggebrecht H, et al. Randomized comparison of strategies for type B aortic dissection: the INvestigation of STEnt Grafts in Aortic Dissection (INSTEAD) trial. Circulation 2009;120:2519-28.

of deep hypothermic circulatory arrest may be necessary for completion of the distal anastomosis.

Surgery is also indicated for complicated type B aortic dissection defined by refractory pain or hypertension, rapid aneurysmal expansion, rupture, or malperfusion syndrome (i.e., end-organ ischemia), whereas medical therapy is the preferred first-line treatment strategy for uncomplicated type B dissection. Dissection location within a previously aneurysmal aortic segment is an anatomical indication for surgical repair. Consideration of aggressive surgical repair also might be given to patients with MFS. Surgery to treat chronic descending thoracic aortic aneurysm is indicated for a maximal dimension ≥5.5 cm. Lower-size thresholds may be appropriate for patients with connective tissue disorders and with accelerated growth rate (≥1 cm/year).

Endovascular Repair

Thoracic endovascular aneurysm repair (TEVAR) (*Figure 9*), percutaneous fenestration, and branch vessel stenting have been evaluated in observational series and randomized trials of patients with acute (or chronic) aortic syndromes. TEVAR has gained increasing acceptance as the treatment of choice for anatomically appropriate type B dissection complicated by malperfusion, dissection progression, impending rupture, hemodynamic instability, or pain refractory to optimal medical therapy. In observational series, morbidity and mortality rates are lower for TEVAR compared with open surgery and similar to those reported for medical therapy in patients with uncomplicated type B dissection.[39,40]

A comprehensive long-term assessment of device-related complications, such as rates of endoleak and stent

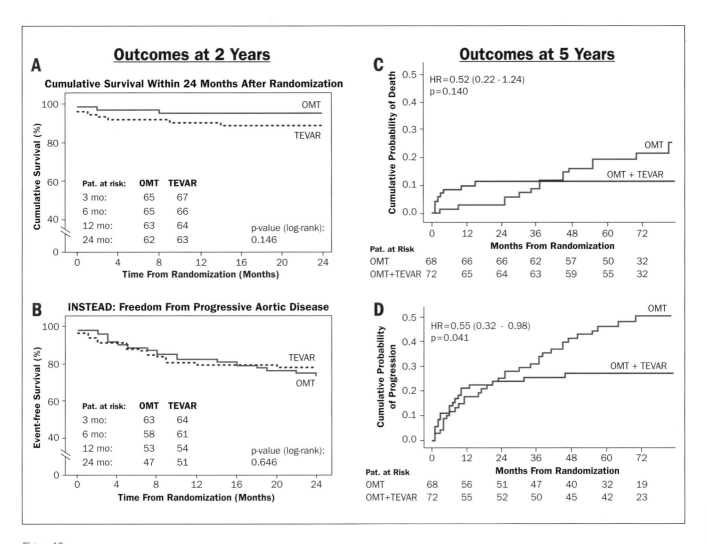

Figure 10

Randomized Comparison of Strategies for Uncomplicated Type B Aortic Dissection

Panels A, B: A randomized trial of 140 patients with stable, uncomplicated type B aortic dissection compared the strategy of TEVAR with OMT versus OMT alone with a primary endpoint of all-cause mortality at 2 years. The TEVAR group did not experience a reduction in all-cause mortality (**panel A**) or freedom from progressive aortic disease (**panel B**) compared with OMT alone at 2 years.

An exploratory analysis of the INSTEAD trial performed 5 years after randomization found no significant difference in all-cause mortality between TEVAR plus OMT versus OMT alone (**panel C**). However, TEVAR was associated with a reduction in the combined endpoint of aortic progression and aortic-related adverse events (**panel D**, aorta-related death, conversion, and ancillary interventions, including a second stent graft procedure, access revision, and peripheral interventions). The curves diverge at 24 months.

HR = hazard ratio; INSTEAD = Investigation of Stent Grafts in Aortic Dissection; OMT = optimal medical management; TEVAR = thoracic endovascular aneurysm repair.

Panels A and B reproduced with permission from Nienaber CA, Rousseau H, Eggebrecht H, et al. Randomized comparison of strategies for type B aortic dissection: the INvestigation of STent Grafts in Aortic Dissection (INSTEAD) trial. Circulation 2009;120:2519-28.

Panels C and D reproduced with permission from Nienaber CA, Kische S, Rousseau H, et al. Endovascular repair of type B aortic dissection: long-term results of the randomized investigation of stent grafts in aortic dissection trial. Circ Cardiovasc Interv 2013;6:407-16.

migration, is needed. It seems unlikely that a randomized trial of TEVAR compared with surgery for complicated acute type B dissection will be performed. The INSTEAD (Investigation of Stent-Grafts in Aortic Dissection) trial enrolled patients with uncomplicated chronic type B dissection and showed no difference in clinical or aortic endpoints at 2 years for patients treated with TEVAR versus those managed medically, although TEVAR was associated with improved survival and morbidity rates at 5 years of follow-up (*Figure 10*). For patients surviving uncomplicated type B dissection, data from retrospective analyses have emerged recently to suggest that intervention in combination with optimal medical therapy is associated with lower mortality and aortic disease progression compared with optimal medical therapy alone at 5 years (*Figure 10*).[41] However, prospective randomized studies in sufficiently sized cohorts remain needed to clarify the long-term role of TEVAR in uncomplicated type B dissection.

Anatomical considerations for TEVAR are reviewed elsewhere. The Society of Thoracic Surgeons has assigned a Class IA recommendation to the use of thoracic stent grafts for repair of acute complicated type B aortic dissection and a Class IC recommendation for acute traumatic transsection.[1,42,43] TEVAR is also recommended for management of complicated PAU disease not responsive to medical therapy or with signs of threatened rupture.

Key Points

- Rapid diagnosis of aortic dissection is critical to a favorable outcome.

- An initial treatment strategy that aims to decrease aortic wall strain by controlling HR and LV contractility (dP/dT) with beta-adrenergic receptor antagonist is advised in AAD.

- Acute type A aortic dissection is a surgical emergency.

- Medical therapy is the preferred first-line treatment strategy for patients with uncomplicated type B aortic dissection.

- Surgery or endovascular intervention may be required in the management of unstable or complicated acute type B aortic dissection, such as in those with malperfusion syndrome or early expansion. In most centers, endovascular therapy including TEVAR has replaced surgery for this indication. The role of TEVAR for uncomplicated type B dissection requires further study.

Prognosis and Recommendations for Aortic Dissection Aftercare

The estimated 1-year survival rate for type A aortic dissection is 60%, although this is contingent upon prompt surgical repair. Hospital mortality rates still approach 25% in many series. The 1-month survival rate for uncomplicated type B aortic dissection is 90%.[37] Many of these patients are self-selected. Factors associated with worse prognosis in acute type B aortic dissection include advanced age, malperfusion syndrome, false lumen partial thrombosis, and surgical treatment. Surgical outcomes are worse because of unavoidable adverse selection bias. Historically, patients with type B dissection referred for surgery have had a greater burden of dissection-related complications and antecedent comorbidities. Patients with maximal thoracic aortic diameter ≥4.0 cm and a patent false lumen have

an increased likelihood of developing subsequent aortic aneurysmal disease.[21,44] Reoperation for late, long-term aortic complications is required in up to a third of survivors.

Routine clinical evaluation at short time intervals and aggressive medical therapy to maintain a target BP of ≤130/80 mm Hg and HR of ≤60 bpm are central to the management of AAS patients following hospital discharge. Beta-receptor antagonists are the mainstay of long-term therapy; other antihypertensive agents commonly are required. Observational data suggest a salutary survival benefit of beta-receptor blockers in survivors of type A dissection and for calcium channel blockers for survivors of type B dissection.[42] In the absence of contraindications, statin therapy typically is initiated owing to the contribution of atherosclerosis to aortic dissection in some patients, especially those with type B disease. To assess for pathological changes in aortic anatomy, patients should undergo serial imaging of the entire aorta at 1, 3, 6, and 12 months following hospital discharge.[37] Patients should be advised against engaging in strenuous exercise, particularly those that involve straining or lifting of heavy weights. These activities are associated with increased aortic wall strain and torsion stress.

Key Points

- Partial thrombosis of the false lumen, false lumen patency, increased age, and malperfusion syndrome are poor prognostic signs in AAD.

- HR and BP control, as well as serial imaging of the entire aorta, is indicated in follow-up for aortic dissection patients surviving to hospital discharge.

Additional Reading

1. Jondeau G, Detaint D, Tubach F, et al. Aortic event rate in the Marfan population: a cohort study. Circulation 2012;125:226-32.

2. Bosner RS, Ranasinghe AM, Loubani M, et al. Evidence, lack of evidence, controversy, and debate in the provision and performance of the surgery of acute type A aortic dissection. J Am Coll Cardiol 2011;58:2455-74.

3. Milewicz KM, Strauss CE, Eagle KA, et al. Correlates of delayed recognition and treatment of acute type A aortic dissection: the International Registry of Acute Aortic Dissection (IRAD). Circulation 2011;124:1911-8.

References

1. Hiratzka LF, Bakris GL, Beckman JA, et al. 2010 ACCF/AHA/ AATS/ACR/ASA/SCA/SCAI/SIR/STS/SVM guidelines for the diagnosis and management of patients with thoracic aortic disease. A report of the American College of Cardiology Foundation/American Heart Association Task Force on Practice

Guidelines, American Association for Thoracic Surgery, American College of Radiology, American Stroke Association, Society of Cardiovascular Anesthesiologists, Society for Cardiovascular Angiography and Interventions, Society of Interventional Radiology, Society of Thoracic Surgeons, and Society for Vascular Medicine. J Am Coll Cardiol 2010;55:e27-e129.

2. DeBakey ME, Beall AC Jr, Cooley DA, et al. Dissecting aneurysms of the aorta. Surg Clin North Am 1966;46:1045-55.

3. Daily PO, Trueblood HW, Stinson EB, Wuerflein RD, Shumway NE. Management of acute aortic dissections. Ann Thorac Surg 1970;10:237-47.

4. Chua M, Ibrahim I, Neo X, Sorokin V, Shen L, Ooi SB. Acute aortic dissection in the ED: risk factors and predictors for missed diagnosis. Am J Emerg Med 2012;30:1622-6.

5. Hagan PG, Nienaber CA, Isselbacher EM, et al. The International Registry of Acute Aortic Dissection (IRAD): new insights into an old disease. JAMA 2000;283:897-903.

6. Olson C, Thelin S, Ståhle E, Ekbom A, Granath F. Thoracic aortic aneurysm and dissection: increasing prevalence and improved outcomes reported in a nationwide population-based study of more than 14,000 cases from 1987 to 2002. Circulation 2006;114:2611-8.

7. Howard DP, Banerjee A, Fairhead JF, Perkins J, Silver LE, Rothwell PM. Population-based study of incidence and outcome of acute aortic dissection and premorbid risk factor control: 10-year results from the Oxford Vascular Study. Circulation 2013;127:2031-7.

8. Keane MG, Pyeritz RE. Medical management of Marfan syndrome. Circulation 2008;117:2802-13.

9. Brooke BS, Habashi JP, Judge DP, et al. Angiotensin II blockade and aortic-root dilation in Marfan's syndrome. N Engl J Med 2008;358:2787-95.

10. Lacro RV, Dietz HC, Sleeper LA, et al. Atenolol versus losartan in children and young adults with Marfan's syndrome. N Engl J Med 2014;371:2061-71.

11. Loeys BL, Dietz HC, Braverman AC, et al. The revised Ghent nosology for the Marfan syndrome. J Med Genet 2010;47:476-85.

12. Guo D, Hasham S, Kuang SQ, et al. Familial thoracic aortic aneurysms and dissections: genetic heterogeneity with a major locus mapping to 5q13-14. Circulation 2001;103:2461-8.

13. Vaughan CJ, Casey M, He J, et al. Identification of a chromosome 11q23.2-q24 locus for familial aortic aneurysm disease, a genetically heterogeneous disorder. Circulation 2001;103:2469-75.

14. Wei LY, Brooke BS, Black JH 3rd. Contemporary management of vascular Ehlers-Danlos syndrome. Curr Opin Cardiol 2011;26:494-501.

15. Pepin M, Schwarze U, Superti-Furga A, et al. Clinical and genetic features of Ehlers–Danlos syndrome type IV, the vascular type. N Engl J Med 2000;342:673-80.

16. Loeys BL, Schwarze U, Holm T, et al. Aneurysm syndromes caused by mutations in the TGF-beta receptor. N Engl J Med 2006;355:788-98.

17. Cameron D. Surgery for congenital diseases of the aorta. J Thorac Cardiovasc Surg 2015;149:S14-7.

18. MacCarrick G, Black JH 3rd, Bowdin S, et al. Loeys-Dietz syndrome: a primer for diagnosis and management. Genet Med 2014;16:576-87.

19. Sorrell VL, Panczyk E, Alpert JS. A new disease: bicuspid aortic valve aortopathy syndrome. Am J Med 2012;125:322-3.

20. Michelena HI, Khanna AD, Mahoney D, et al. Incidence of aortic complications in patients with bicuspid aortic valves. JAMA 2011;306:1104-12.

21. Maron BA, O'Gara PT. Pathophysiology, clinical evaluation, and medical management of aortic dissection. In: Creager M, Beckman JA, Loscalzo J, eds. Vascular Medicine: A Companion to Braunwald's Heart Disease. 2nd ed. Philadelphia: Saunders; 2013:687-96.

22. Braverman AC. Acute aortic dissection: clinician update. Circulation 2010;122:184-8.

23. Ketenci B, Enc Y, Ozay B, et al. Perioperative type I aortic dissection during conventional coronary artery bypass surgery: risk factors and management. Heart Surg Forum 2008;11:E231-6.

24. Stanger O, Schachner T, Gahl B, et al. Type A aortic dissection after nonaortic cardiac surgery. Circulation 2013;128:1602-11.

25. Elefteriades JA. Natural history of thoracic aortic aneurysm: indications for surgery, and surgical versus nonsurgical risks. Ann Thorac Surg 2002;74:S1877-80.

26. Pape LA, Tsai TT, Isselbacher EM, et al. Aortic diameter ≥5.5 cm is not a good predictor of type A aortic dissection: observations from the International Registry of Acute Aortic Dissection (IRAD). Circulation 2007;116:1120-7.

27. Tsai TT, Evangelista A, Nienaber CA, et al. Partial thrombosis of the false lumen in patients with acute type B aortic dissection. N Engl J Med 2007;357:349-59.

28. Harris KM, Strauss CE, Eagle KA, et al. Correlates of delayed recognition and treatment of acute type A aortic dissection: the International Registry of Acute Aortic Dissection (IRAD). Circulation 2011;124:1911-8.

29. Evangelista A, Mukherjee D, Mehta RH, et al. Acute intramural hematoma of the aorta: a mystery in evolution. Circulation 2005;111:1063-70.

30. Kang DH, Song JK, Song MG, et al. Clinical and echocardiographic outcomes of aortic intramural hemorrhage compared with acute aortic dissection. Am J Cardiol 1998;81:202-6.

31. Nienaber CA, von Kodolitsch Y, Petersen B, et al. Intramural hemorrhage of the thoracic aorta. Diagnostic and therapeutic implications. Circulation 1995;92:1465-72.

32. Strauss C, Harris K, Hutchison S, et al. Time is life: early mortality in type A acute aortic dissection: insights from the IRAD Registry. J Am Coll Cardiol 2013;61:1159-107.

33. Bossone E, Rampoldi V, Nienaber CA, et al. Usefulness of pulse deficit to predict in-hospital complications and mortality in patients with acute type A aortic dissection. Am J Cardiol 2002;89:851-5.

34. Rogers AM, Hermann LK, Booher AM, et al. Sensitivity of the aortic dissection detection risk score, a novel guideline-based tool for identification of acute aortic dissection at initial presentation: results from the International Registry of Acute Aortic Dissection. Circulation 2011;123:2213-8.

35. Erbel R, Alfonso F, Boileau C, et al. Diagnosis and management of aortic dissection. Eur Heart J 2001;22:1642-81.

36. Macura KJ, Szarf G, Fishman EK, Bluemke DA. Role of computed tomography and magnetic resonance imaging in assessment of acute aortic syndromes. Semin Ultrasound CT MR 2003;24:232-54.

37. Suzuki T, Isselbacher EM, Nienaber CA, et al. Type-selective benefits of medications in treatment of acute aortic dissection (from the International Registry of Acute Aortic Dissection [IRAD]). Am J Cardiol 2012;109:122-7.

38. Mastroroberto P, Onorati F, Zofrea S, Renzulli A, Indolfi C. Outcome of open and endovascular repair in acute type B aortic dissection: a retrospective and observational study. J Cardiothorac Surg 2010;5:23.

39. Luebke T, Brunkwall J. Outcome of patients with open and endo-vascular repair in acute complicated type B aortic dissection: a systematic review and meta-analysis of case series and compara-tive studies. J Cardiovasc Surg (Torino) 2010;51:613-32.

40. Kim KH, Moon IS, Park JS, Koh YB, Ahn H. Nicardipine hydro-chloride injectable phase IV open-label clinical trial: study on the anti-hypertensive effect and safety of nicardipine for acute aortic dissection. J Int Med Res 2002;30:337-45.

41. Cohen O, Odim J, De la Zerda D, et al. Long-term experience of gir-dling the ascending aorta with Dacron mesh as definitive treatment for aneurysmal dilation. Ann Thorac Surg 2007;83:S780-4.

42. Svensson LG, Kouchoukos NT, Miller DC, et al. Expert consensus document on the treatment of descending thoracic aortic disease using endovascular stent-grafts. Ann Thorac Surg 2008;85:S1-41.

43. Nienaber CA, Rousseau H, Eggebrecht H, et al. Randomized comparison of strategies for type B aortic dissection: the IN-vestigation of STEnt Grafts in Aortic Dissection (INSTEAD) trial. Circulation 2009;120:2519-28.

44. Yeh CH, Chen MC, Wu YC, Chu JJ, Lin PJ. Risk factors for de-scending aortic aneurysm formation in medium-term follow-up of patients with type A aortic dissection. Chest 2003;124:989-95.

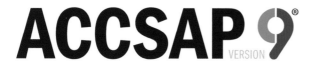

ACCSAP 9

Adult Clinical Cardiology Self-Assessment Program

Book 6
Vascular Diseases

PERIPHERAL ARTERY DISEASE

Editor:

Patrick T. O'Gara, MD, MACC
This author has nothing to disclose.

Lower Extremity Peripheral Artery Disease

Introduction

Peripheral artery disease (PAD) is primarily the result of atherosclerosis in the arteries of the lower extremities, and is frequently associated with atherosclerosis in all vascular distributions. As a result, the presence of PAD confers a significant risk of cardiovascular morbidity and mortality, primarily as a result of stroke (from cerebrovascular atherosclerosis) and myocardial infarction (MI) (from coronary atherosclerosis). The early recognition of PAD therefore provides a unique opportunity to identify individuals at high risk for adverse cardiovascular events, treat systemic atherosclerosis, tailor preventive therapy, and improve cardiovascular outcomes.

Epidemiology

The prevalence of PAD increases with advancing age, affecting nearly 8.5 million individuals in the United States. The prevalence of PAD is 5.8% among the population above the age of 40, essentially doubling with each decade of life thereafter. Disease prevalence is also associated with ethnicity, affecting predominantly non-Hispanic whites, but—in older age groups—PAD is identified in African Americans at rates nearly two to three times greater than others.[1,2] Worldwide, the incidence of PAD is on the rise, with a 23.5% increase between 2000-2010, and more than 202 million people affected.[3]

In addition to increasing age, the risk factors responsible for PAD are similar to those for coronary artery disease: diabetes, tobacco use, hypertension, and dyslipidemia have the strongest impact. Both diabetes and tobacco use each confer a three- to fourfold increase in the risk of developing PAD. Unlike coronary disease, however, in population-based studies, the prevalence of PAD is equal in men and women.[4,5]

Key Point

- PAD is highly prevalent, particularly with advancing age, affecting nearly 8.5 million Americans, 19% of the population over the age of 70, and more than 202 million persons worldwide.

Diagnosis

Most often, PAD is either clinically silent or is manifest as intermittent claudication (IC). "Classic" IC was originally described by Rose, and is characterized by:

- Pain that is brought on by exertion (walking)

- Pain that is relieved within 10 minutes of rest

- Pain that does not occur at rest

Of note, only 10-30% of patients with PAD experience classic IC symptoms. Many complain of leg weakness or heaviness.

Douglas E. Drachman, MD, FACC

Consultant Fees/Honoraria: Abbott Vascular, Corindus Vascular Robotics, St. Jude Medical; Data Safety Monitoring Board: PLC Medical Systems, Prairie Education & Research Cooperative.

Learner Objectives

Upon completion of this module, the reader will be able to:

1. Recognize that peripheral arterial disease (PAD) is a marker for systemic atherosclerosis and is significantly associated with adverse cardiovascular events.

2. Identify the common risk factors predisposing individuals to PAD.

3. Discuss the appropriate evaluation and treatment of patients with PAD.

Grade	Category	Clinical Symptoms
0	0	Asymptomatic
I	1	Mild claudication
	2	Moderate claudication
	3	Severe claudication
II	4	Ischemic rest pain
	5	Minor tissue loss
III	6	Major tissue loss

Table 1
Rutherford Classification Scheme for Peripheral Arterial Disease

Stage	Clinical Symptoms
I	Asymptomatic
IIa	Mild claudication
IIb	Moderate to severe claudication
III	Rest pain
IV	Ulcer or gangrene

Table 2
Fontaine Classification Scheme

It is estimated that 25-60% of patients with PAD are asymptomatic.

The two most common classification schemes for PAD are the Rutherford and Fontaine classifications (*Tables 1, 2*).

In more severe cases, PAD may progress to include pain at rest, skin breakdown or ulceration, and gangrene, three hallmark findings of "critical limb ischemia" (CLI). Patients with advanced PAD may describe a pain, ache, or numbness in the leg at rest, worsened with elevation of the leg, and relieved with dependent positioning, such as dangling the leg off the edge of the bed.

Physical examination for PAD may disclose:

- Diminished or absent pulses

- Bruits (carotid, supraclavicular, abdominal, femoral)

- Muscle atrophy

- Dependent rubor and elevation pallor of the feet

- Signs of CLI: hair loss, smooth/shiny skin, dystrophic nails, coolness, pallor or cyanosis of the foot

In evaluating patients with possible PAD, it is important to differentiate between other processes with similar symptom profiles. Degenerative disc disease or spinal stenosis may manifest similar leg pain with exertion ("pseudoclaudication"). In some instances, patients may describe pain that persists while standing still, or pain that is relieved while continuing to walk, leaning forward over a shopping cart; such symptoms are less characteristic of PAD and more likely indicative of pseudoclaudication. Diabetic neuropathy, deconditioning, and muscular strain are other entities that may be difficult to distinguish from PAD.

Perhaps the most useful and cost-effective tool to diagnose PAD is the ankle-brachial index (ABI) (*Figure 1*). The study is performed by applying a blood pressure cuff to the calf, then measuring blood pressure at the ankle using a continuous-wave Doppler probe. The higher of the dorsalis pedis or posterior tibial artery pressures is recorded as the ankle pressure. The process is repeated with the cuff on the biceps and the Doppler on the brachial artery, quantifying the brachial pressure. The ABI is then calculated by dividing the ankle pressure by the higher of the two brachial pressures. In healthy individuals, the ankle pressure should be higher than the brachial pressure, with a resulting ABI of 0.9-1.3. If the ankle pressure is more than 10% lower than the brachial pressure (i.e., ABI <0.9), this serves as the diagnosis for PAD. In cases of severe PAD, potentially with rest pain, the ABI is typically less than 0.4. In cases where the lower extremity arteries are calcified and noncompressible, as may be the case in disease states such as diabetes and renal failure, the ABI may be elevated; if the ABI is greater than 1.3, the ankle vessels are deemed "noncompressible," which is also suggestive of vascular disease.

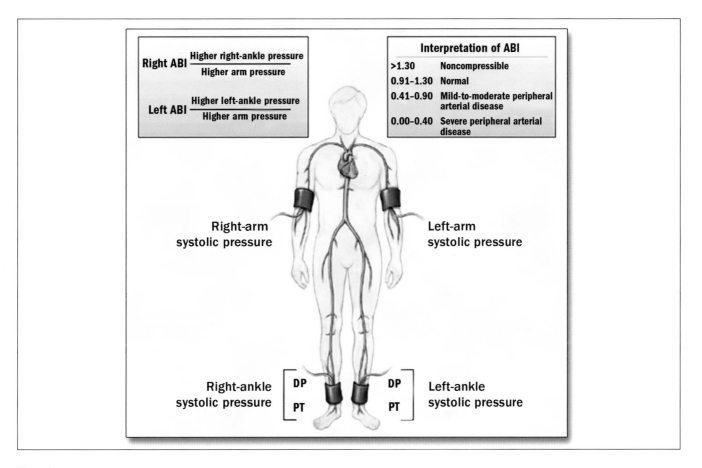

Figure 1
The Ankle-Brachial Index

ABI = ankle-brachial index; DP = dorsalis pedis; PT = posterior tibial.

Modified from Hiatt WR. Medical treatment of peripheral arterial disease and claudication. N Engl J Med 2001;344:1608-21.

In patients who have a history consistent with IC, but have an unremarkable physical examination and resting ABI, exercise treadmill testing with ABI may help discriminate between pseudoclaudication and IC. According to the standard protocol, patients walk on a treadmill at 2.0 mph with a 12% grade for a maximum of 5 minutes. In the Gardner/Hiatt protocol, the speed is held constant, but the grade is gradually increased during the period of exertion. In both protocols, the ABI is measured at rest and post-exercise. The addition of exercise serves several purposes:

- The increased demand for flow and the peripheral vasodilatation that occurs with exertion may unmask or accentuate the hemodynamic impact of an arterial stenosis, which may be subtle on resting ABI.

- The exercise program provides a universal "yardstick" to evaluate functional capacity, and may be a handy measure of performance pre- and post-revascularization.

- Exercise may uncover occult coronary disease or angina pectoris.

For its roles in identifying patients with PAD, discriminating claudication from pseudoclaudication, and for assessing functional capacity, exercise treadmill testing with ABI receives a Class I indication in the American College of Cardiology/American Heart Association (ACC/AHA) Practice Guidelines for the Management of Patients with PAD.[6]

Segmental limb pressures, analogous to the ABI, assess the blood pressure at sequentially more distal loci along the length of the leg: thigh, calf, ankle, transmetatarsal, and digits. Identifying the location in the leg where the blood pressure abruptly diminishes relative to the brachial pressure, one may determine the level at which the arterial obstruction occurs.

Pulse volume recording (plethysmography) provides a noninvasive assessment of the arterial waveform at sequential loci along the leg. Identifying areas where the amplitude of the waveform becomes diminished, and where the contour of the waveform becomes blunted and widened, may provide insight into the presence and severity of obstruction at the immediately adjacent arterial segments.

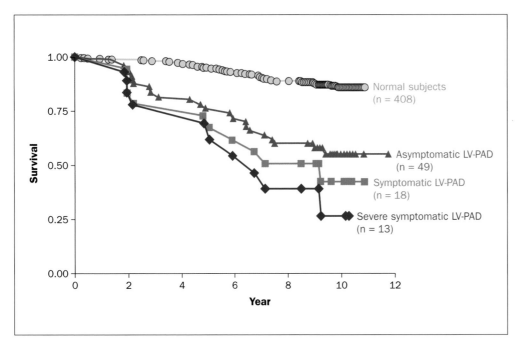

Figure 2
More Severe PAD Confers Higher Risk of Morbidity and Mortality, Primarily Due To Adverse Cardiovascular Events

LV-PAD = large vessel peripheral arterial disease.

Reproduced with permission from Criqui MH, Langer RD, Fronek A, et al. Mortality over a period of 10 years in patients with peripheral arterial disease. N Engl J Med 1992;326:381-6.

Noninvasive anatomic imaging studies, including duplex ultrasonography, magnetic resonance angiography, and computed tomography angiography, may provide an exquisite roadmap of the vasculature if revascularization is being considered. These studies, however, are not the first-line approach to making the diagnosis of PAD.

Invasive angiography represents the "gold standard" for anatomic imaging. In cases where an arterial stenosis is of indeterminate severity, hemodynamic evaluation may be considered by measuring a pressure gradient across the lesion; the utility of invasive pressure wire assessment is being validated in various arterial distributions. Intraluminal anatomic visualization also may be performed with intravascular ultrasound; at present, optical coherence tomography has not been extensively studied in the periphery, and invasive angioscopy remains primarily a research tool.

Natural History

In the majority of patients diagnosed with PAD, the outcomes with respect to the limb are, ironically, less morbid than the systemic manifestations of panvascular atherosclerosis. Specifically, for patients who present with claudication, the vast majority (73%) will have stable symptoms over the ensuing 5 years. While 16% may have progressive claudication, only 7% will require surgical revascularization, and 4% will require amputation.[7] Predictors of progressive PAD include diabetes, tobacco use, ABI <0.5, or ankle pressure <70 mm Hg.

In contrast, identification of PAD in the context of claudication confers a 25-30% 5-year mortality in those over 55 years old; 75% of the deaths are a result of cardiovascular causes. An additional 20% of individuals with IC will suffer nonfatal cardiovascular events (MI, stroke).[8]

Moreover, the more severe the clinical manifestation of PAD (i.e., severe claudication or rest pain with skin breakdown and ulceration vs. no symptoms), the worse the overall risk of adverse cardiovascular events (*Figure 2*).[1] Of note, worse outcomes are not a result of limb-specific events, but rather a result of elevated rates of stroke, MI, and cardiovascular death. In essence, a higher atherosclerotic burden in the legs, manifested as worse claudication, predicts higher atherosclerotic burden in the heart and cerebral vasculature, with an increased burden of associated morbidity and mortality.

Key Point

- The diagnosis of PAD confers a 25-30% 5-year risk of cardiovascular death and an additional 20% risk of nonfatal major adverse cardiovascular events.

Public Awareness

A major impediment to the appropriate treatment of PAD is the fact that the disease remains under-recognized by the public and that the clinical implications of the diagnosis are underappreciated, even within the medical community. The mortality of PAD exceeds that of breast cancer or Hodgkin's disease, and is just below that of colon cancer (*Figure 3*).[9]

In a telephone survey of 2,501 Americans above the age of 50, only 26% were "very" or "somewhat" familiar with PAD. A higher percentage of individuals surveyed recognized cystic fibrosis (29%), Lou Gehrig's disease (amyotrophic lateral sclerosis [ALS], 36%), and multiple sclerosis (42%). Comparatively, however, while PAD affects nearly 9 million individuals in the United States, cystic fibrosis affects 30,000, ALS affects 20,000, and multiple

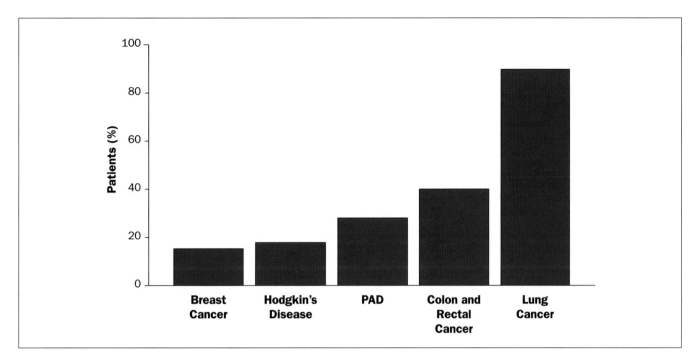

Figure 3

Five-Year Mortality of Peripheral Arterial Disease vs. Common Types of Cancer

PAD = peripheral arterial disease.

Reproduced with permission from Criqui MH. Systemic atherosclerosis risk and the mandate for intervention in atherosclerotic peripheral arterial disease. Am J Cardiol 2001;88:43J-47J.

sclerosis affects 300,000. The need for improved public awareness of PAD, given its high prevalence and profound morbidity, is paramount.[10]

Treatment

Therapy for PAD is focused on prevention of cardiovascular events, amelioration of claudication symptoms, and prevention of skin breakdown, wound formation, or infection. A multidisciplinary task force was established to provide guidelines for the management of patients with PAD; a brief summary of their recommendations is noted in the following section.[6]

The primary method to prevent adverse cardiovascular events in patients with PAD is through a focus on risk factor modification.

Smoking Cessation
Cigarette smoking is the risk factor most strongly correlated with PAD. It follows that smoking cessation offers significant opportunity to improve limb as well as general cardiovascular outcomes. In one study, smoking cessation improved mean treadmill walking distance by 40% at 10 months compared with patients who failed to quit smoking.[11] In two studies of patients undergoing vascular surgery, smoking cessation (or reduction) improved 3-year survival from 40% to 65-67%.[12,13]

Lipid-Lowering Therapy
In the 2013 ACC/AHA Guideline on the Treatment of Blood Cholesterol to Reduce Atherosclerotic Cardiovascular Risk in Adults, PAD is considered equivalent to atherosclerotic cardiovascular disease. Accordingly, there is a Class I (Level of Evidence A) recommendation for secondary prevention in PAD patients using high-intensity statin therapy (atorvastatin 40-80 mg daily or rosuvastatin 20-40 mg daily) for individuals who are 75 or younger. Those above 75, or those who are not candidates for high-intensity statin, should be treated with a moderate-intensity statin.[14] Among the 6,748 individuals with PAD in the Heart Protection Study, the use of simvastatin reduced mortality by 12%, vascular mortality by 17%, adverse coronary events by 24%, and stroke by 27% at a mean follow-up of 5 years. In addition, lipid lowering may improve symptoms of claudication and extend walking times.[15]

Glycemic Control in Diabetes
In recent years, the perspective on glycemic control in patients with type 2 diabetes mellitus—including those with PAD—has shifted from achieving a specific glycemic target to one that is individualized to the patient. With a paucity of comparative effectiveness data identifying a single superior approach, and with data indicating that aggressive glycemic control may cause harm, recommendations are now focused on patient-centered goals.[16]

Antiplatelet Therapy

Antiplatelet therapy receives a Class I recommendation in the ACC/AHA Guidelines for Prevention of Adverse Cardiovascular Events in Patients With PAD. The Antithrombotic Trialists' Collaboration evaluated the findings from 42 clinical trials, which included outcomes for 9,214 patients with PAD, to define the impact of antiplatelet therapy on cardiovascular events. Patients with PAD who received antiplatelet therapy had a nearly 25% reduction in the rate of stroke, MI, or cardiovascular death when compared with patients who received placebo. Because the majority of these studies involved the use of aspirin, the ACC/AHA guidelines support the use of aspirin as a Class I recommendation (Level of Evidence A).[17] In the CAPRIE (Clopidogrel versus Aspirin in Patients at Risk for Ischemic Events) study, more than 19,000 patients with a history of ischemic stroke, MI, or symptomatic PAD were randomized to treatment with either aspirin or clopidogrel. Individuals assigned to clopidogrel treatment had a relative reduction in the composite endpoint of MI, stroke, or vascular death of 8.7% compared with those taking aspirin alone; this effect was more pronounced in the subgroup of patients with PAD, where the composite endpoint was reduced by 23.8%. In light of these findings, the ACC/AHA PAD guidelines and the TASC-II (Trans-Atlantic Society-II) guidelines support the use of clopidogrel monotherapy as an alternative to aspirin in patients with PAD (Class I, Level of Evidence B).[6,7]

Protease-Activated Receptor-1 (PAR-1) Inhibition

The PAR-1 inhibitor vorapaxar reduced adverse limb events in patients with PAD enrolled in the TRA2°P-TIMI 50 (Trial to Assess the Effects of Vorapaxar in Preventing Heart Attack and Stroke in Patients With Atherosclerosis) clinical trial. This prospective, randomized controlled trial examined the impact on the composite endpoint of cardiovascular death, MI, or stroke in 26,449 subjects who received vorapaxar or placebo control. In a subgroup analysis of 3,787 subjects with PAD, there was no significant difference in the composite primary endpoint (11.3% vs. 11.9%, p = 0.53), but the rate of acute limb ischemia requiring hospitalization (2.3% vs. 3.9%; hazard rate [HR] 0.58; 95% confidence interval [CI], 0.39-0.86; p = 0.006) and the need for PAD revascularization (18.4% vs. 22.2%; HR 0.84; 95% CI, 0.73-0.97; p = 0.017) were significantly lower in individuals allocated to vorapaxar therapy, albeit with an elevated bleeding risk (7.4% vs. 4.5%; HR 1.62; 95% CI, 1.21-2.18; p = 0.001). Vorapaxar has been approved by the Food and Drug Administration (FDA) for reduction of thrombotic cardiovascular events in patients with a history of MI or PAD.[18]

Antihypertensive Therapy

Control of hypertension is recommended in all patients with PAD. Targets for blood pressure reduction remain the subject of debate. In the HOPE (Heart Outcomes Prevention Evaluation) trial, use of ramipril reduced the risk of MI by 22% in patients with PAD.[19] Beta-blockers were once thought to worsen claudication; in large studies, however, their use has not been associated with more severe or limiting symptoms.

Foot Care

Patients with PAD should receive meticulous foot care on a routine basis in order to minimize the risk of skin breakdown and/or the development of infection.

Exercise Therapy for Claudication

Symptoms of claudication may most commonly be managed with conservative therapy. Supervised exercise constitutes the cornerstone of treatment for IC. In a meta-analysis of 21 studies of supervised walking programs, the mean walking distance to onset of claudication was increased by two blocks—a 180% improvement—compared with baseline after a walking program. The absolute walking distance was improved by three blocks (120%) compared with baseline.[20]

Home-based walking programs also have been shown to be beneficial. In one study, 194 patients with PAD were randomized to a home-based walking program or control. Those who pursued the home-based program significantly increased their mean 6-minute walking distance compared to those in the control group with commensurate improvement in Walking Impairment Questionnaire outcomes.[21]

A variety of mechanisms have been proposed to explain how exercise improves claudication, including: vascular angiogenesis ("collateral" vessel development), increased exercise pain tolerance, improved muscle energy metabolism, improved endothelial function, decreased inflammation and free radical formation in muscle, and reduced blood viscosity and red blood cell aggregation.

In the CLEVER (Claudication: Exercise Vs. Endoluminal Revascularization) trial, 111 patients with claudication and aortoiliac PAD were randomized to treatment with a supervised exercise program, endovascular therapy with stenting, or optimal medical care (including cilostazol pharmacotherapy). At 6 months, the primary endpoint—improvement in peak walking time—was greatest for those enrolled in a supervised exercise program (5.8 +/- 4.6 minutes more than baseline), intermediate for those who underwent stenting (3.7 +/- 4.9), and least for those treated with optimal medical care (1.2 +/- 2.6). Interestingly, the quality-of-life improvement—measured using the Walking Impairment Questionnaire and the Peripheral Artery Questionnaire—was improved with both supervised exercise and stenting (compared with optimal medical care), but was more improved with stenting than with exercise. While this study demonstrates the important roles for exercise and endovascular therapy in the management of patients with aortoiliac disease, the generalizability of the findings warrants further study. The trial involved a small and highly select cohort of patients, which may not reflect real-world clinical scenarios. The discrepancy between the treadmill and quality-of-life outcomes may cloud the trial's potential impact on practice. Supervised exercise programs are not currently reimbursed for patients with PAD under Medicare guidelines. Longer-term follow-up will be required to assess the durability of these treatment strategies.[22]

The ERASE (Endovascular Revascularization and Supervised Exercise) trial, while similar in concept, had several significant differences from the CLEVER trial. ERASE randomized 212 patients with claudication and aortoiliac or femoropopliteal artery disease to treatment with supervised exercise therapy alone, or supervised exercise therapy plus endovascular therapy. The primary endpoint evaluated the improvement in maximum walking distance at 12 months between the two groups. Supervised exercise improved walking distance from 285m to 1240m (955m improvement), while endovascular therapy plus exercise improved walking distance significantly more, from 264m to 1501m (1237m improvement, 99% CI, 60-505m). Furthermore, the addition of endovascular therapy to supervised exercise significantly improved pain-free walking distance and subjective measures of quality of life, including VascuQOL score and SF-36 questionnaire data. Unlike in CLEVER, where supervised exercise alone and endovascular therapy alone were compared head-to-head, ERASE demonstrated that endovascular therapy *plus exercise* resulted in superior outcomes to supervised exercise alone.[23]

Pharmacotherapy for Claudication

Medical therapy may also improve symptoms of claudication. The current FDA-approved therapies for claudication include cilostazol and pentoxifylline. Cilostazol is a phosphodiesterase inhibitor (PDE-3), which promotes vasodilatation and inhibits platelet aggregation. In clinical trials, cilostazol improved IC distance after 12 weeks of therapy compared with placebo (from baseline 71.2m to post-treatment 112.5m, compared with 77.7m to 84.6m, respectively; p = 0.007); absolute claudication distance was also improved (141.9m to 231.7m, compared with 168.6m to 152.1m, respectively; p = 0.002). Cilostazol is generally perceived to be more effective than pentoxifylline, but bears a black-box warning from the FDA for use in patients with congestive heart failure.[24] Cilostazol receives a Class I indication (Level of Evidence A) to reduce symptoms of claudication and improve walking distance in patients with lower extremity PAD.[6] As noted previously in the CLEVER trial, cilostazol—administered to those patients receiving optimal medical care—was inferior to either supervised exercise programs or endovascular therapy.[22] Pentoxifylline was shown to provide only modest improvement in absolute walking distance compared with placebo control in a meta-analysis of 11 clinical trials.[25] Pentoxifylline receives only a Class IIb indication for therapy for IC in the ACC/AHA PAD and TASC-II guidelines.

Endovascular Therapy

In select individuals, revascularization also may be considered for the treatment of PAD. In cases of severe limb ischemia, such as CLI where the viability of the limb is threatened, the indication for revascularization may be clear. Perfusion to the foot is typically very poor, with ankle pressures <40 mm Hg and toe pressures <30 mm Hg. Without revascularization, loss of skin integrity may confer risk for infection, gangrene, and irreparable tissue loss. There is debate as to whether such patients are better treated with endovascular therapy or with surgical revascularization. Endovascular options are minimally invasive, and confer lower risk of perioperative stress and significant adverse cardiovascular events when compared with surgery. Surgical bypass was long held as the gold standard treatment for patients with CLI. The comparative effectiveness of various revascularization strategies has been evaluated in recent randomized controlled trials.

In the BASIL (Bypass versus angioplasty in severe ischaemia of the leg) trial, 452 patients were randomized to an initial strategy of bypass surgery or endovascular treatment with angioplasty (not stenting) for infrainguinal disease. No between-group difference in the primary composite endpoint of amputation-free survival at 3 years was found.[26]

In trials of endovascular management of superficial femoral artery (SFA) disease, angioplasty has been compared with stenting. In one study of 104 patients, those who underwent stenting had a 24% restenosis rate (angiographically determined) at 6 months compared with 43% in those who underwent angioplasty alone (p < 0.05). By duplex ultrasonography at 12 months, the restenosis rates were 27% and 63%, respectively (p = 0.01). Walking distance was greater at 1 year in those patients receiving stents (387m) compared with those who underwent angioplasty alone (267m, p = 0.04). These findings suggest that endovascular therapy for the SFA using nitinol self-expanding stents may provide greater durability than angioplasty alone.[27]

The use of drug-eluting stents (DES) may improve the durability of endovascular treatment in the femoropopliteal segment. In the Zilver PTX study, patients with femoropopliteal PAD were randomized to treatment with primary DES (n = 236) or primary angioplasty (n = 238). If primary angioplasty resulted in a suboptimal outcome (such as flow-limiting dissection), those individuals underwent secondary randomization to treatment with provisional bare metal stent (BMS, n = 59) or DES (n = 61). At 2 years, primary patency was 74.8% (primary DES) versus 26.5% (angioplasty, p = 0.02), and 83.4% (provisional DES) versus 64.1% (provisional BMS, p < 0.01) with higher sustained clinical benefit in patients treated with DES.[28]

Drug-coated balloon (DCB) therapy also has been demonstrated to improve durability of outcomes in femoropopliteal artery intervention. In the IN.PACT SFA (Drug-Coated Balloon versus Standard Percutaneous Transluminal Angioplasty for the Treatment of Superficial

Femoral and/or Popliteal Peripheral Artery Disease) trial, 331 patients with femoropopliteal PAD were enrolled (2:1) to treatment with DCB versus angioplasty alone. At 2 years, primary patency with DCB (78.9%) was superior to angioplasty (50.1%, p < 0.001) with commensurately lower rates of clinically driven target lesion revascularization (9.1% vs. 28.3%, respectively, p < 0.001).[29] In the LEVANT 2 (Lutonix Paclitaxel-Coated Balloon for the Prevention of Femoropopliteal Restenosis 2) trial, a different DCB was shown to have superior primary patency (65.2% vs. 52.6%, p = 0.02) at 1 year when compared with conventional angioplasty in 476 patients with symptomatic femoropopliteal PAD.[30]

The optimal method of revascularization for infrapopliteal disease has been controversial. In these relatively narrow-caliber vessels, atherosclerotic disease is often very diffuse and is frequently associated with CLI; the lesions are often heavily calcified and recalcitrant to endovascular techniques. Over the past 2 decades, however, the development of narrow-caliber angioplasty balloons and more sophisticated guide wires have allowed significant improvement in transcatheter techniques. In a prospective, nonrandomized case series of 235 sequential patients undergoing tibioperoneal angioplasty, 95% of patients were treated successfully with endovascular technique, with limb salvage rates of 91% among survivors at mean follow-up of 34 months. While restenosis rates may be high following tibioperoneal angioplasty (12 month primary patency rates of 22- 92% in meta-analyses), the rates of limb salvage may remain excellent (50-92%, although mostly 80-90% in the same series).[31,32] Recently, the 3-year outcomes of the OLIVE registry were reported, examining infrainguinal endovascular therapy for CLI. This prospective, multicenter registry included 314 individuals who had a 55.2% rate of amputation-free survival, 88.4% freedom from major adverse limb events, and wound-free survival in 49.6%.[33] In concept, re-establishing "straight line flow" from the heart to the foot may enable wound healing in critical limb ischemia, even if the durability of current below-knee endovascular treatment approaches remains limited.

Although many novel interventional therapies have been developed to facilitate endovascular intervention, to date, none has been shown in rigorous fashion to provide superior outcomes in terms of amputation-free survival when compared with angioplasty alone. Such technologies include: rotational atherectomy, orbital atherectomy, directional atherectomy, laser atherotomy, cutting balloon atherotomy, cryoplasty, and infrapopliteal stenting. Whether DES or DCB may improve outcomes in CLI, and whether there may be opportunity to leverage new technologies, such as bioresorbable vascular scaffolds, remains to be seen.

Surgical Therapy

Surgical bypass typically is reserved for patients with limb-threatening ischemia or disabling claudication. Considerations for surgery include patient-specific risks for adverse cardiovascular events, and a careful preoperative evaluation is required. Adequate conduit must be available for bypass; in many circumstances, autologous venous conduit is ideal, but in some cases, prosthetic material may need to be substituted. Arterial anatomy—with consideration of adequate "inflow" as well as reasonable "outflow"—must be ascertained (*Table 3*).

Key Points

- Treatment of PAD includes a focus on prevention of stroke and MI:

  ○ Smoking cessation

  ○ High-intensity statin therapy in patients <75 years; moderate-intensity statin therapy in those >75 years, or those who are not candidates for high-intensity statin therapy

  ○ Glycemic control, with strategy and A1c target tailored to the patient

  ○ Antihypertensive therapy

  ○ Antiplatelet therapy

  ○ Consideration of adjunctive PAR-1 inhibitor therapy in patients with low bleeding risk

- For severe limb ischemia, revascularization therapy is required. Optimal approach varies as a function of clinical presentation, lesion location and type, and patient comorbidities.

Acute Limb Ischemia

Acute limb ischemia (ALI) is an uncommon manifestation of PAD, but carries substantial risk of morbidity and mortality. ALI is characterized by the "6 Ps" of pain, pallor, pulselesssness, paresthesia, paralysis, and poikilothermia (coolness), and may represent imminent threat to the extremity. Mechanistically, ALI often may result from acute embolic arterial occlusion. Emboli may originate from a central cardiac source, such as in the setting of atrial fibrillation, or from a more proximal aneurysm, such as in the aorta or popliteal artery. In-situ thrombosis on a severely stenotic plaque, especially in the context of a hypercoagulable state, may also result in ALI.

The onset of ALI represents a true emergency, equivalent to a "leg attack." If the limb remains ischemic for more than 6 hours, permanent ischemic sensory and motor

Arterial Distribution	Revascularization Technique	Primary Patency	Notes
Iliac	Aortobifemoral bypass (Dacron)	87-91% at 5 years[1,2]	Mortality 3.3-4.6%[1,2]
	Iliac PTA	55-85% at 3 years[3]	>90% acute success rate[4,5]
	Iliac stent	77% at 4 years (stenosis) 61% at 4 years (occlusion)[5]	96% acute success[5]
SFA	Above-knee femoral popliteal bypass: SVG	74-76% at 5 years[1,6-9]	
	Above-knee femoral popliteal bypass: PTFE	39-52% at 5 years[1,6-9]	
	Femoropopliteal PTA	55% at 5 years (stenosis) 42% at 5 years (occlusion)[1]	
	Femoropopliteal stent	66% at 3 years (stenosis) 64% at 3 years (occlusion)[1]	
	Femoropopliteal DCB	78.9% at 2 years	IN.PACT SFA[10]
	Femoropopliteal DCB	65.2% at 1 year	LEVANT-2[11]
	Femoropopliteal DES	74.8% at 2 years	Zilver PTX[12]
Infrapopliteal	Femoral-tibiopedal bypass: SVG	60% assisted 5-year patency[1]	
	Femoral-tibiopedal bypass: PTFE	35% assisted 5-year patency[1]	
	Infrapopliteal PTA	22-92% at 1 year 9-51% at 2 years[13]	

Table 3

Patency Rates Following Revascularization Techniques in Each Lower Extremity Vascular Territory

The term "primary patency" refers to the freedom from repeat revascularization, where revascularization is driven either by recurrent symptoms, or evidence of significant recurrent stenosis. The term "assisted patency" refers to a vessel which has required repeat revascularizations to remain patent.

DCB = drug-coated balloon; DES = drug-eluting stent; PTA = percutaneous transluminal angioplasty; PTFE = polytetrafluoroethylene; SFA = superficial femoral-popliteal artery; SVG = saphenous vein graft.

References:

1. Norgren L, Hiatt WR, Dormandy JA, Nehler MR, Harris KA, Fowkes FG, on behalf of the TASC II Working Group. Inter-society consensus for the management of peripheral arterial disease (TASC II). J Vasc Surg 2007;45 Suppl S:S5-67.

2. de Vries SO, Hunink MG. Results of aortic bifurcation grafts for aortoiliac occlusive disease: a meta-analysis. J Vasc Surg 1997;26:558-69.

3. Tetteroo E, van der Graaf Y, Bosch JL, et al. Randomised comparison of primary stent placement versus primary angioplasty followed by selective stent placement in patients with iliac-artery occlusive disease. Dutch Iliac Stent Trial Study Group. Lancet 1998;351:1153-9.

4. Rooke TW, Hirsch AT, Misra S, et al. Management of patients with peripheral artery disease (compilation of 2005 and 2011 ACCF/AHA guideline recommendations): a report of the American College of Cardiology Foundation/ American Heart Association Task Force on Practice Guidelines. J Am Coll Cardiol 2013;61:1555-70.

5. Bosch JL, Tetteroo E, Mali WP, Hunink MG. Iliac arterial occlusive disease: cost-effectiveness analysis of stent placement versus percutaneous transluminal angioplasty. Dutch Iliac Stent Trial Study Group. Radiology 1998;208:641-8.

6. Green RM, Abbott WM, Matsumoto T, et al. Prosthetic above-knee femoropopliteal bypass grafting: five-year results of a randomized trial. J Vasc Surg 2000;31:417-25.

7. AbuRahma AF, Robinson PA, Holt SM. Prospective controlled study of polytetrafluoroethylene versus saphenous vein in claudicant patients with bilateral above knee femoropopliteal bypasses. Surgery 1999;126:594-601; discussion 601-2.

8. Johnson WC, Lee KK. A comparative evaluation of polytetrafluoroethylene, umbilical vein, and saphenous vein bypass grafts for femoral-popliteal above-knee revascularization: a prospective randomized Department of Veterans Affairs cooperative study. J Vasc Surg 2000;32:268-77.

9. Klinkert P, van Dijk PJ, Breslau PJ. Polytetrafluoroethylene femorotibial bypass grafting: 5-year patency and limb salvage. Ann Vasc Surg 2003;17:486-91.

10. Laird JR, Schneider PA, Tepe G, et al., on behalf of IN.PACT SFA Trial Investigators. Durability of treatment effect using a drug-coated balloon for femoropopliteal lesions: 24-month results of IN.PACT SFA. J Am Coll Cardiol 2015;66:2329-38.

11. Rosenfield K, Jaff MR, White CJ, et al., on behalf of the LEVANT 2 Investigators. Trial of a paclitaxel-coated balloon for femoropopliteal artery disease. N Engl J Med 2015;373:145-53.

12. Dake MD, Ansel GM, Jaff MR, et al., on behalf of Zilver PTX Investigators. Sustained safety and effectiveness of paclitaxel-eluting stents for femoropopliteal lesions: 2-year follow-up from the Zilver PTX randomized and single-arm clinical studies. J Am Coll Cardiol 2013;61:2417-27.

13. Lipsitz EC, Veith FJ, Ohki T. The value of subintimal angioplasty in the management of critical lower extremity ischemia: failure is not always associated with a rethreatened limb. J Cardiovasc Surg (Torino) 2004;45:231-7.

loss may ensue. Following diagnosis of ALI, an infusion of unfractionated heparin should be initiated immediately, while plans for revascularization are underway.

Invasive angiography, with plans to pursue endovascular revascularization, is the standard first-line approach. Catheter-directed thrombolysis with tissue-plasminogen activator may be considered if the thrombus burden is substantial. Suction thrombectomy and rheolytic thrombectomy are adjunctive endovascular approaches to reduce thrombus burden and may be used in conjunction with angioplasty and stenting. In some cases, surgical thrombectomy or bypass may be required.

Following reperfusion, the limb should be monitored closely for edema and tissue swelling causing compartment syndrome. In severe cases, swelling—constrained within fascial compartments of the leg—may lead to permanent nerve injury with sensory and motor loss if surgical fasciotomy is not performed.

Conclusion

PAD serves as a marker for systemic atherosclerosis and confers a high risk for major adverse cardiovascular events. Treatment is focused on prevention of adverse cardiovascular events, amelioration of IC symptoms, and limb salvage. Through improved public awareness and physician recognition of PAD, there is dramatic opportunity to improve cardiovascular outcomes in this highly prevalent disease state.

References

1. Allison MA, Ho E, Denenberg JO, et al. Ethnic-specific prevalence of peripheral arterial disease in the United States. Am J Prev Med 2007;32:328-33.

2. Mozaffarian D, Benjamin EJ, Go AS, et al., on behalf of the American Heart Association Statistics Committee and Stroke Statistics Subcommittee. Heart disease and stroke statistics--2015 update: a report from the American Heart Association. Circulation 2015;131:e29-e322.

3. Fowkes FG, Rudan D, Rudan I, et al. Comparison of global estimates of prevalence and risk factors for peripheral artery disease in 2000 and 2010: a systematic review and analysis. Lancet 2013;382:1329-40.

4. Hirsch AT, Criqui MH, Treat-Jacobson D, et al. Peripheral arterial disease detection, awareness, and treatment in primary care. JAMA 2001;286:1317-24.

5. Selvin E, Erlinger TP. Prevalence of and risk factors for peripheral arterial disease in the United States: results from the National Health and Nutrition Examination Survey, 1999-2000. Circulation 2004;110:738-43.

6. Rooke TW, Hirsch AT, Misra S, et al. Management of patients with peripheral artery disease (compilation of 2005 and 2011 ACCF/AHA guideline recommendations): a report of the American College of Cardiology Foundation/American Heart Association Task Force on Practice Guidelines. J Am Coll Cardiol 2013;61:1555–70.

7. Norgren L, Hiatt WR, Dormandy JA, Nehler MR, Harris KA, Fowkes FG, on behalf of the TASC II Working Group. Inter-society consensus for the management of peripheral arterial disease (TASC II). J Vasc Surg 2007;45 Suppl S:S5-67.

8. Weitz JI, Byrne J, Clagett GP, et al. Diagnosis and treatment of chronic arterial insufficiency of the lower extremities: a critical review. Circulation 1996;94:3026-49.

9. Criqui MH. Systemic atherosclerosis risk and the mandate for intervention in atherosclerotic peripheral arterial disease. Am J Cardiol 2001;88:43J-47J.

10. Hirsch AT, Murphy TP, Lovell MB, et al., on behalf of the Peripheral Arterial Disease Coalition. Gaps in public knowledge of peripheral arterial disease: the first national PAD public awareness survey. Circulation 2007;116:2086-94.

11. Quick CR, Cotton LT. The measured effect of stopping smoking on intermittent claudication. Br J Surg 1982;69 Suppl:S24-6.

12. Faulkner KW, House AK, Castleden WM. The effect of cessation of smoking on the accumulative survival rates of patients with symptomatic peripheral vascular disease. Med J Aust 1983;1:217-9.

13. Lassila R, Lepäntalo M. Cigarette smoking and the outcome after lower limb arterial surgery. Acta Chir Scand 1988;154:635-40.

14. Stone NJ, Robinson JG, Lichtenstein AH, et al. 2013 ACC/AHA guideline on the treatment of blood cholesterol to reduce atherosclerotic cardiovascular risk in adults: a report of the American College of Cardiology/American Heart Association Task Force on Practice Guidelines. J Am Coll Cardiol 2014;63:2889-934.

15. Heart Protection Study Collaborative Group. MRC/BHF Heart Protection Study of cholesterol lowering with simvastatin in 20,536 high-risk individuals: a randomised placebo-controlled trial. Lancet 2002;360:7-22.

16. Inzucchi SE, Bergenstal RM, Buse JB, et al. Management of hyperglycemia in type 2 diabetes: a patient-centered approach: position statement of the American Diabetes Association (ADA) and the European Association for the Study of Diabetes (EASD). Diabetes Care 2012;35:1364-79.

17. Antithrombotic Trialists' Collaboration. Collaborative meta-analysis of randomised trials of antiplatelet therapy for prevention of death, myocardial infarction, and stroke in high risk patients. BMJ 2002;324:71-86.

18. Bonaca M, Creager M, Olin J, et al. Vorapaxar reduces peripheral revascularization regardless of the number of diseased territories: insights from the TRA2P–TIMI 50 TRIAL. J Am Coll Cardiol. 2013;61(10_S):. doi:10.1016/S0735-1097(13)62018-5.

19. Effects of ramipril on cardiovascular and microvascular outcomes in people with diabetes mellitus: results of the HOPE study and MICRO-HOPE substudy. Heart Outcomes Prevention Evaluation Study Investigators. Lancet 2000;355:253-9.

20. Gardner AW, Poehlman ET. Exercise rehabilitation programs for the treatment of claudication pain: a meta-analysis. JAMA 1995;274:975-80.

21. McDermott MM, Liu K, Guralnik JM, et al. Home-based walking exercise intervention in peripheral artery disease: a randomized clinical trial. JAMA 2013;310:57-65.

22. Murphy TP, Cutlip DE, Regensteiner JG, et al., on behalf of CLEVER Study Investigators. Supervised exercise versus primary stenting for claudication resulting from aortoiliac peripheral artery disease: six-month outcomes from the claudication: exercise versus endoluminal revascularization (CLEVER) study. Circulation 2012;125:130-9.

23. Fakhry F, Spronk S, van der Laan L, et al. Endovascular re-vascularization and supervised exercise for peripheral artery disease and intermittent claudication: a randomized clinical trial. JAMA 2015;314:1936-44.

24. Dawson DL, Cutler BS, Meissner MH, Strandness DE Jr. Cilostazol has beneficial effects in treatment of intermittent claudication: results from a multicenter, randomized, prospective, double-blind trial. Circulation 1998;98:678-86.

25. Hood SC, Moher D, Barber GG. Management of intermittent claudication with pentoxifylline: meta-analysis of randomized controlled trials. CMAJ 1996;155:1053-9.

26. Adam DJ, Beard JD, Cleveland T, et al., on behalf of the BASIL trial participants. Bypass versus angioplasty in severe ischaemia of the leg (BASIL): multicentre, randomised controlled trial. Lancet 2005;366:1925-34.

27. Schillinger M, Sabeti S, Loewe C, et al. Balloon angioplasty versus implantation of nitinol stents in the superficial femoral artery. N Engl J Med 2006;354:1879-88.

28. Dake MD, Ansel GM, Jaff MR, et al., on behalf of Zilver PTX Investigators. Sustained safety and effectiveness of paclitaxel-eluting stents for femoropopliteal lesions: 2-year follow-up from the Zilver PTX randomized and single-arm clinical studies. J Am Coll Cardiol 2013;61:2417-27.

29. Laird JR, Schneider PA, Tepe G, et al., on behalf of IN.PACT SFA Trial Investigators. Durability of treatment effect using a drug-coated balloon for femoropopliteal lesions: 24-month results of IN.PACT SFA. J Am Coll Cardiol 2015;66:2329-38.

30. Rosenfield K, Jaff MR, White CJ, et al., on behalf of the LEVANT 2 Investigators. Trial of a paclitaxel-coated balloon for femoropopliteal artery disease. N Engl J Med 2015;373:145-53.

31. Dorros G, Jaff MR, Dorros AM, Mathiak LM, He T. Tibioperoneal (outflow lesion) angioplasty can be used as primary treatment in 235 patients with critical limb ischemia: five-year follow-up. Circulation 2001;104:2057-62.

32. Lipsitz EC, Veith FJ, Ohki T. The value of subintimal angioplasty in the management of critical lower extremity ischemia: failure is not always associated with a rethreatened limb. J Cardiovasc Surg (Torino) 2004;45:231-7.

33. Iida O, Nakamura M, Yamauchi Y, et al., on behalf of the OLIVE Investigators. 3-year outcomes of the OLIVE Registry, a prospective multicenter study of patients with critical limb ischemia: a prospective, multi-center, three-year follow-up study on endovascular treatment for infra-inguinal vessel in patients with critical limb ischemia. JACC Cardiovasc Interv 2015;8:1493-502.

Upper Extremity Peripheral Artery Disease

Introduction

Upper extremity peripheral artery disease (PAD) is far less prevalent than lower extremity PAD, comprising approximately 5% of all limb ischemia. While lower extremity PAD is primarily atherosclerotic in etiology, upper extremity PAD is also commonly associated with several other disease states.

Consequently, methods for the evaluation and treatment of upper extremity PAD may vary, reflecting the unique character and pathophysiology of the lesions associated with different underlying disease processes. The assessment and management of patients with upper extremity PAD are dependent on an understanding of the etiologic factors and a tailored approach to treatment.

Key Points

- Upper extremity PAD is far less common than lower extremity PAD.

- While the symptoms from various upper extremity arterial disease states may bear similarities, the underlying disease processes are unique entities and warrant specific attention and tailored evaluation and management approaches.

Epidemiology

Upper extremity PAD may be grouped into two major categories: 1) those disease that affect the large arteries, which lie between the aorta and the wrist, and 2) those that affect the small arteries, which lie distal to the wrist.

Large-vessel upper extremity PAD may be subcategorized further as:

- Vasculopathy, including atherosclerotic disease (the most common etiologic factor) and vasculitis.

- Vascular and neurovascular entrapment (thoracic outlet syndrome [TOS]).

- Embolic disease.

- Aneurysmal disease.

Small-vessel upper extremity PAD may reflect several disease processes, such as collagen vascular disease with associated vasculitis; hematologic disease, including hypercoagulable states and blood dyscrasias; Buerger's disease (thromboangiitis obliterans [TAO]); and embolic disease.

Vasospastic disease—Raynaud's disease in particular—may exist independently or in conjunction with other large- or small-vessel upper extremity PAD.[1]

Douglas E. Drachman, MD, FACC
Consultant Fees/Honoraria: Abbott Vascular, Corindus Vascular Robotics, St. Jude Medical; Data Safety Monitoring Board: PLC Medical Systems, Prairie Education & Research Cooperative.

Learner Objectives

Upon completion of this module, the reader will be able to:

1. Evaluate the history and physical findings of patients presenting with upper extremity peripheral artery disease (PAD).
2. Determine the appropriate evaluation to identify the underlying cause and manifestations of upper extremity PAD.
3. Recognize that upper extremity PAD may be one manifestation of significant, underlying systemic disease.
4. Establish an appropriate treatment plan for patients with upper extremity PAD.

Diagnosis

History

While the history and physical examination play a critical role in the identification of upper extremity PAD, the cardinal manifestations—which most commonly result from stenosis of the inflow to the arm (the subclavian artery), occlusion of the small outflow vessels in the hand, or vasospasm—may be similar across many disease processes. Inflow disease typically is characterized by arm discomfort or fatigue with exertion (claudication). Outflow disease may result in symptoms focused in the hand and fingers, including rest pain, discoloration, cold intolerance, and ulceration. In addition, many disease processes may provoke vasospasm and the predominant symptoms may result from this superimposed disorder.

The history may prove particularly valuable, however, in identifying other comorbidities that may be associated with upper extremity PAD, including autoinflammatory disorders, atherosclerosis with other systemic manifestations, or hematologic disorders. A history of exposure to toxic substances, drugs, medications, or tobacco may shed light on the cause of upper extremity PAD. A history of repetitive trauma, such as the use of crutches or the occupational use of a hammer or jackhammer, should be considered in patients presenting with arm or hand symptoms suggestive of axillary artery aneurysm or hypothenar hammer syndrome, respectively.

Physical Examination

The physical examination should include visual inspection to assess for digital ulceration, discoloration, livedo reticularis or signs of distal embolization, dystrophic nails, signs of repetitive trauma, or other manifestations of an associated connective tissue disorder, such as telangiectasias in the nail fold associated with scleroderma. A comprehensive pulse examination should be performed to evaluate the time of arrival and the amplitude and contour of the pulse, as well as palpate for any aneurysmal dilatation, paying particular attention to the artery in the supraclavicular fossa and axilla.

Auscultation for bruits should be performed in the supraclavicular fossa and at the base of the carotid arteries with the arm at rest and with provocative maneuvers (abduction and external rotation) to exclude dynamic impingement or entrapment of the subclavian artery in TOS (Adson's maneuver). An Allen's test, performed by occluding flow in both the radial and ulnar arteries, having the patient clench and relax the fist multiple times, releasing either the radial or ulnar artery, and watching for return of capillary perfusion throughout the hand, may establish whether arterial flow across the palmar arch is intact. Performance of an Allen's test is required before transradial artery access for cardiac catheterization.

Other Studies

Appropriately selected noninvasive studies may provide significant data to complement the history and physical examination and to help discriminate between the various etiologies of upper extremity PAD.

Segmental limb pressures and pulse volume recordings may provide significant insight into the location and hemodynamic impact of stenoses in upper extremity PAD. Cuff pressures are measured at the brachial artery, upper forearm, wrist, and finger. Pressures are compared with the corresponding loci in the contralateral arm. A decrement of >15 mm Hg between two sequential loci in an arm suggests that a significant stenosis exists between them. Likewise, a discrepancy of ≥15 mm Hg between left and right brachial artery pressures suggests subclavian stenosis in the arm with the lower pressure.

The amplitude and waveform of the pulse volume recording may demonstrate if there is impediment to flow: blunted waveform or diminution of the contour from triphasic to biphasic to monophasic may represent successively more severe stenosis proximal to the site of pulse volume recording. When assessing for TOS, pulse volume recordings may be assessed at rest, then with provocative maneuvers, to evaluate for dynamic arterial impingement.

Duplex scans using color flow technique may identify sites of stenosis and provide insight into stenosis severity. Duplex scanning also may demonstrate the presence of aneurysmal disease.

Radiography may be useful to assess for the presence of a cervical rib in patients with TOS. Computed tomographic angiography and magnetic resonance angiography (MRA) may provide highly detailed delineation of the arterial anatomy. MRA with diffusion-weighted imaging also may demonstrate edema in the vessel wall in cases of inflammatory vasculitis, such as Takayasu arteritis. Invasive angiography remains the "gold standard" method to identify vascular anatomy.

In cases of dynamic arterial obstruction, such as TOS, provocative maneuvers should be performed during imaging to identify entrapment/impingement of vascular structures.

In patients in whom the diagnosis of Raynaud's disease is suspected, cold water immersion may be considered, but the limited sensitivity and specificity of this assessment make definitive diagnosis difficult to establish.[2]

Laboratory assessment may be useful in identifying comorbid conditions that are associated with the development of upper extremity PAD. Routine chemistries and complete blood count should be performed. When evaluating for inflammatory or collagen vascular disease states, erythrocyte sedimentation rate (ESR),

C-reactive protein (CRP), antinuclear antibody, and rheumatoid factor may provide further insights. In patients with suspected embolic disease or with secondary Raynaud's disease, a hypercoagulability workup may be helpful. Echocardiography also may be helpful to establish a structural or cardiac source of embolism. Patients with atherosclerotic subclavian artery disease should have a lipid profile.

Natural History

Subclavian Artery Stenosis

Atherosclerosis is the most common cause of subclavian artery disease. The left subclavian artery (LSA) is affected three- to fourfold more frequently than the right subclavian artery (RSA). The stenosis most often occurs at the ostium or in the proximal portion of the vessel, proximal to the origins of the left vertebral and internal mammary arteries. Most subclavian stenoses are asymptomatic. In cases of severe stenosis, symptoms of claudication may be noted in the ipsilateral limb, typically presenting as fatigue and discomfort with exertion, which are alleviated with rest.

When stenosis of the LSA is severe and is proximal to the origin of the left vertebral artery, collateral perfusion to the left arm may develop via retrograde flow from the posterior cerebral circulation to the left vertebral artery, termed "subclavian steal." Many individuals with subclavian steal may remain asymptomatic and may never develop vertebrobasilar insufficiency unless there is other disease that interferes with perfusion of the posterior circulation, such as contralateral carotid or vertebral stenosis or diseased or hypoplastic posterior communicating arteries.

When the reversal of flow in the left vertebral artery prompts symptoms, it is known as "subclavian steal syndrome." Symptoms may include dizziness, vertigo, ataxia, visual disturbance, and syncope. In patients who have undergone coronary artery bypass graft surgery employing a left internal mammary artery (LIMA) graft, subclavian steal syndrome may provoke "steal" of coronary flow from the LIMA graft, resulting in coronary ischemia and angina. Patients with high grade proximal LSA stenosis may also develop postoperative angina in the absence of a "steal" phenomenon.

On physical examination, a patient with subclavian artery stenosis typically has at least a 15 mm Hg decrement in brachial artery systolic pressure compared with the contralateral arm; the brachial, radial, and ulnar pulses may be diminished (and delayed) compared with the contralateral arm; and a supraclavicular bruit often may be appreciated on auscultation.

Assessment for subclavian steal may be performed using duplex ultrasound. Severity of stenosis may be identified on interrogation of the subclavian artery, and flow in the left vertebral artery may be examined. Of note, in patients with symptoms of subclavian steal syndrome, flow in the left vertebral artery may be retrograde, bidirectional, or even anterograde at rest. Typically, following arm ergometry or after provoking hyperemia of the arm by inflating a blood pressure cuff to suprasystolic levels for 5 minutes and then relaxing the cuff, flow in the left vertebral artery likely will become biphasic or reversed in cases with subclavian steal.

Additionally, subclavian steal physiology may be documented with invasive angiography by injection of contrast into the contralateral vertebral or carotid circulation. Phase contrast MRA may demonstrate reversal of flow in the left vertebral artery.

In a longitudinal study of 1,778 patients from two vascular laboratory cohorts and one general population cohort, 8.8% of patients were found to have subclavian stenosis (mean age 68 years). Among these patients, the presence of subclavian stenosis served as a marker for increased risk of cardiovascular disease mortality (hazard ratio [HR], 1.50; p = 0.05).[3] Additionally, in the Framingham Heart Study, an interarm systolic blood pressure difference of 10 mm Hg or greater was associated with an increased risk of adverse cardiovascular events (HR, 1.38; 95% confidence interval [CI], 1.09-1.75).[4]

Since subclavian stenosis is often asymptomatic and serves as an indicator of increased risk for adverse events from atherosclerosis, the cornerstone of therapy for subclavian stenosis involves risk factor modification (see module on *Lower Extremity Peripheral Artery Disease* in this chapter).

In cases where a subclavian artery stenosis is symptomatic, however, options for treatment include bypass surgery and endovascular therapy. Bypass surgery, most commonly a polytetrafluoroethylene (PTFE) bypass graft from the common carotid artery to the subclavian artery, was the previous "gold standard" for treatment of symptomatic subclavian stenosis. Complications with surgery occur in up to 11-13% of patients, including stroke in 3% and death in 2%. Other severe complications include injury of the thoracic duct, resulting in chylothorax; cranial nerve injury; recurrent (graft) stenosis; and graft infection.[5,6]

The evolution of endovascular technologies and techniques, however, has altered the treatment of subclavian artery stenoses. In the largest single-center experience, 170 patients with subclavian or innominate artery stenosis underwent endovascular treatment with stent insertion (177 lesions). Technical success was achieved in 98.3% with no deaths, one stroke (0.6%), and 3-year target lesion revascularization rate of 14.6%.[7] While revascularization is nearly always reserved for individuals with symptomatic stenosis, one instance where asymptomatic subclavian stenosis may warrant treatment is in management of disease prior to the use of the ipsilateral internal mammary artery for coronary artery bypass surgery.[8,9]

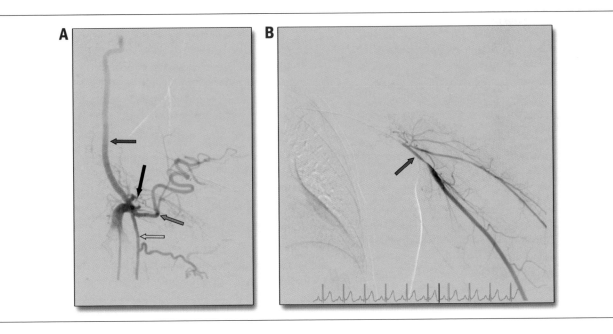

Figure 1

Digital Subtraction Angiography of the Left Subclavian (Panel A) and Left Axillary Arteries (Panel B) in a 33-Year-Old Man With Takayasu Arteritis

Note the total occlusion of the left subclavian artery (black arrow) just beyond the origins of the left vertebral (red arrow) and left internal mammary arteries (yellow arrow, **panel A**). The green arrow in **panel A** indicates a large collateral vessel, delivering flow to the reconstitution of the distal vessel in the axillary artery (blue arrow, **panel B**).

Images provided courtesy of Kenneth Rosenfield, MD, Massachusetts General Hospital, Boston, MA.

In cases where the subclavian artery is totally occluded, the endovascular technique may be technically challenging and in some cases not feasible. These patients remain candidates for bypass surgery. Otherwise, whenever technically feasible, subclavian stenting is now viewed as the first-line approach.[10]

Innominate artery stenosis is far less common than subclavian stenosis. The assessment and treatment strategies are analogous.

Giant Cell Arteritis (Temporal Arteritis)

Giant cell arteritis (GCA) constitutes a systemic, inflammatory condition that primarily affects Caucasian, Northern European women >60 years.[11] While the hallmark symptoms of disease are headache, jaw claudication, and transient monocular blindness, extracranial manifestations may commonly include vascular inflammation of the upper extremity vessels, primarily the axillary, subclavian, and brachial arteries. Unlike atherosclerotic disease, which tends to affect primarily the proximal portion of the subclavian artery, GCA tends to provoke more diffuse disease, and may progress from stenosis to occlusion or aneurysm.[12]

In patients with GCA, the ESR typically is elevated (>50 sec) and the C-reactive protein (CRP) level is elevated with 100% sensitivity. In one study, the combination of elevated ESR and CRP was predictive of GCA with 97% specificity.[13] There is commonly an association with

anticardiolipin antibody, particularly in patients with active disease.[14] The diagnosis of GCA may be confirmed by temporal artery biopsy, though diagnostic yield can be less than anticipated.

Treatment of GCA with corticosteroids and immunosuppressive therapy is primarily systemic. Surgical bypass or endovascular therapy may be considered for cases of severe limb ischemia, although it is highly preferable to perform revascularization in a relatively quiescent phase of the disease.

Takayasu Arteritis

Compared with GCA, Takayasu arteritis occurs predominantly in younger women (mean age of onset in the mid-20s) and is more common in those of Asian or South American descent.[15,16] The arteritis may involve the subclavian and axillary arteries (*Figure 1*). As with GCA, therapy is typically directed systemically with corticosteroids or methotrexate if the inflammation is not responsive to steroids. Antiplatelet and lipid-lowering therapies also are recommended.

Revascularization may be considered in cases of severe upper extremity ischemia or severe subclavian steal. The lesions of Takayasu arteritis may be very fibrotic and therefore may be very recalcitrant to endovascular therapy; restenosis rates of 26% have been described following percutaneous angioplasty (PTA).[17,18]

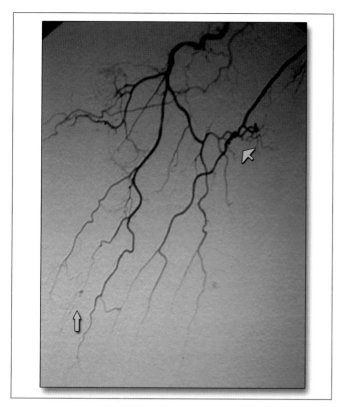

Figure 2

Digital Subtraction Angiography of the Right Hand in a Patient With Thromboangiitis Obliterans (Buerger's Disease)

Note the occlusion of the distal digital arteries (narrow arrow) and the corkscrew collateral at the distal ulnar artery (broad arrow head).

Image provided courtesy of Michael R. Jaff, DO, Massachusetts General Hospital, Boston, MA.

Buerger's Disease (Thromboangiitis Obliterans)
Buerger's disease is primarily a disease of small and medium arteries and veins, including the palmar, radial, and ulnar arteries in the upper extremity. Patients with Buerger's disease often present with distal, digital symptoms, including pain, stigmata of thrombotic distal vascular occlusion, and ulceration. Pathophysiologically, the disease is characterized by thrombosis of the small and medium vessels, where the thrombi are highly cellular with inflammatory cells and leukocyte infiltration, disproportionate to the degree of inflammation in the vessel wall.

Angiography discloses thrombotic occlusion of the small and medium vessels with corkscrew collaterals, primarily due to ectatic, irregular development of the vasa vasorum (*Figure 2*).

Buerger's disease is intimately linked with tobacco use. The disease occurs more commonly in men than women and almost always presents before the age of 45 years. The cornerstone of therapy is absolute cessation of tobacco use. Unfortunately, the rate of relapse to smoking is very high, and the corresponding rate of tissue loss is 40%.[19]

Other Small Vessel Disease States
Many other systemic conditions may result in obstruction of the small vessels in the upper extremity. Connective tissue disorders such as the CREST syndrome, scleroderma, systemic lupus erythematosus, and rheumatoid arthritis may promote small vessel vasculitis. In these cases, the vasculitis is managed by treating the underlying systemic inflammatory condition, typically with immunosuppressant therapy or corticosteroids.

Hypercoagulable states, such as antiphospholipid antibody syndrome, lupus anticoagulant, heparin-induced thrombocytopenia, and others, may result in occlusion of small vessels. Treatment may include systemic anticoagulation or other antithrombotic therapy. Blood dyscrasia, such as cryoglobulinemia (hepatitis C) and myeloproliferative disorders, also may lead to vasculitis and occlusion of small vessels. Therapy typically is focused on treatment of the underlying systemic illness.

Thoracic Outlet Syndrome
TOS results from compression of the nerve or vascular structures that exit the superior outlet of the thorax. The brachial plexus exits the scalene triangle (between the anterior and middle scalene muscles) and then passes over the first rib and under the clavicle through the costoclavicular space (*Figure 3*). The brachial plexus is joined in the costoclavicular space by the subclavian artery and vein. The nerve and vascular structures especially may be subjected to compression in the costoclavicular space in patients who have a cervical first rib.[20]

Most cases (95%) of TOS involve impingement of the brachial plexus, and 5% involve vascular compromise. The symptoms of TOS often are provoked by arm activity, particularly when the arm is raised above the head, and characterized by ache and fatigue. Many cases of TOS are characterized by symptoms due to superimposed Raynaud's disease. TOS cases with arterial involvement are rare but may have severe consequences. Initially, symptoms may be mild due to gradual development of collaterals. Over time, stenosis and poststenotic dilatation may occur, and symptoms may worsen abruptly due to thrombosis proximally or distal embolization.[21]

Evaluation of patients with TOS should include bilateral arm blood pressures and a pulse examination at rest and with provocative maneuvers. Adson's maneuver involves abduction and external rotation of the arm, and is potentiated further by turning the head in the opposite direction and having the patient take a deep breath. During the maneuver, the ipsilateral arm pulses should diminish. Auscultation may also disclose a bruit due to dynamic subclavian artery compression during provocative maneuvers. TOS maneuvers may be positive in 15% of patients with no symptoms; conversely, maneuvers may be negative in patients with known TOS.[20,21]

Radiography should be performed to exclude a cervical first rib. Angiography should be performed in patients with

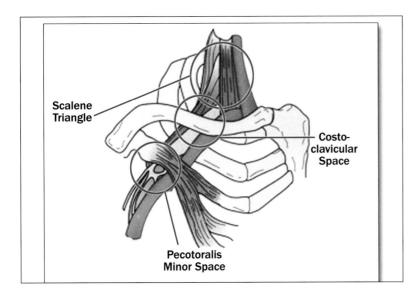

Figure 3
Anatomy of Thoracic Outlet Syndrome

Thoracic outlet syndrome results from compression of the nerve and/or vascular structures that exit the superior outlet of the thorax. The brachial plexus exits the *scalene triangle* (between the anterior and middle scalene muscles) and then passes over the first rib and under the clavicle through the *costoclavicular space*. The brachial plexus is joined in the costoclavicular space by the subclavian artery and vein. The nerve and vascular structures especially may be subjected to compression in the costoclavicular space in patients who have a cervical first rib.

Adapted from Sanders RJ and Annest SJ. Thoracic outlet and pectoralis minor syndromes. Semin Vasc Surg 2014;27:86-117.

TOS who have developed peripheral emboli or in patients being considered for surgery.

Therapy for TOS includes physical therapy to address posture and minimize nerve and vascular impingement in the thoracic outlet. Surgery may be considered, particularly in cases of a cervical rib, where rib resection may reduce vessel entrapment in the costoclavicular space. In a recent case series, surgery was performed in 19 limbs in 18 patients with arterial TOS: 8 had critical ischemia (5 acute and 3 acute-on-chronic) and 11 had claudication. All surgeries included decompression of the thoracic outlet; 13 required arterial reconstruction and 7 included treatment for distal arterial emboli. One patient underwent treatment for chylothorax 2 weeks after surgery; and one patient required treatment for bypass graft thrombosis at 4 months.[22]

Complications of Transradial Arterial Access

Over the past 2 decades, and particularly over the past 5-10 years, there has been a tremendous surge in the adoption of transradial arterial access for cardiovascular procedures. While in the United States the adoption rate has increased from 1.3% in 2007 to 16% in 2012, many other countries employ transradial access in >30-40% of procedures.[23,24]

Clinical trials have demonstrated that transradial access is associated with lower rates of bleeding and other vascular complications compared with transfemoral access. In the management of patients with ST elevation myocardial infarction (STEMI), transradial access is associated with a reduction in the rate of death. The most common access site complications following transradial access include[23,25]:

- Radial artery occlusion (RAO, 2-18%).

  ○ Usually clinically silent, given redundant vascular supply to the hand via the ulnar artery and palmar arch, although rare case reports of hand ischemia exist. RAO avoidance strategies include systemic anticoagulation, antivasospasm medications, patent hemostasis, and case selection.

- Radial artery spasm (5-30%).

- Bleeding (1-2%).

- Radial perforation (0.1-1%).

- Aseptic granuloma (reaction to lubricious sheath coating, rare).

- Arteriovenous fistula (rare).

- Pseudoaneursym (rare).

- Nerve injury (rare).

Aneurysm

The natural history, prognosis, and treatment strategies for aneurysms in the upper extremity vary based on the location and etiology of the lesion. In the subclavian artery, aneurysms may develop from a variety of different causes. In TOS, recurrent impingement of the subclavian artery may lead to stenosis with poststenotic dilatation. In many cases, release of vessel impingement—most often resection of a cervical rib—may promote remodeling and resolution of the poststenotic dilatation. In cases where aneurysmal dilatation continues to progress, resection of the aneurysm with placement of an interposition graft (autologous saphenous vein) is required.

Subclavian artery aneurysms may also be caused by atherosclerosis or trauma. In certain lesions, PTFE-covered stent grafts may be considered for aneurysm exclusion using endovascular technique. In subclavian artery aneurysms due to inflammatory vasculitis (giant cell arteritis, Takayasu arteritis), treatment is focused on management of the underlying inflammation with corticosteroids or immunosuppressive therapy.

In patients with an aberrant RSA (arteria lusoria), which is a congenital vascular anomaly in which the RSA arises from the aorta distal to the take-off of the LSA, 60% of patients may develop aneurysmal dilatation of the vessel

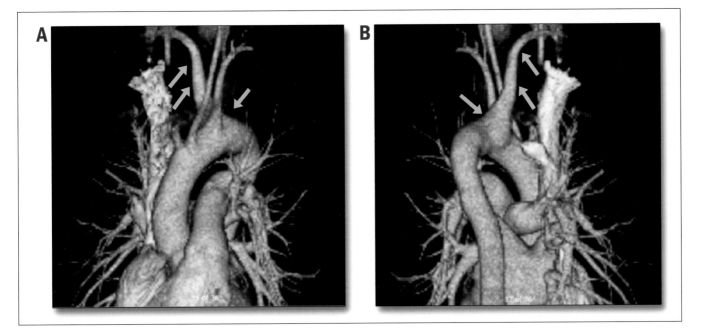

Figure 4

Computed Tomography Angiography of Kommerell Diverticulum

Note the aberrant, distal origin of the right subclavian artery (single arrow), with aneurysmal dilatation. The course of the vessel, crossing from the left side of the aortic arch to the right, is indicated with two arrows. An anterior projection is shown in **panel A**; a posterior projection is shown in **panel B**. The outpunching at the origin of the aberrant right subclavian artery represents the Kommerell diverticulum, and is better seen in the posterior projection.

Image provided courtesy of David M. Dudzinski, MD, Massachusetts General Hospital, Boston, MA.

origin, termed a Kommerell diverticulum (*Figure 4*). The artery courses between the esophagus and the spine; in certain cases, vascular impingement of the esophagus or of the recurrent laryngeal nerve may lead to dysphagia and hoarseness, termed dysphagia lusoria. Patients with a Kommerell diverticulum and dysphagia lusoria are prone to aneurysmal rupture and may benefit from prophylactic surgical repair.[26,27] A recent case series described the management of 24 patients with aberrant RSA, seven of whom had a Kommerell diverticulum. All seven patients required surgical repair: three for symptoms (43%) and four for aneurysmal change in the aorta (57%). Of the 10 patients in the case series who required surgery, there was one postoperative death (10%).[28]

Axillary artery aneurysms most commonly are due to traumatic injury. The most common mechanism is the use of crutches, causing repetitive axillary trauma. Other repetitive trauma, such as the occupational use of a hammer or jackhammer or involvement in professional sports with repetitive aggressive motion of the wrist and arm (baseball pitching, golf), may result in hypothenar hammer syndrome, characterized by ulnar arterial injury with stenosis or aneurysm formation.

Raynaud's Disease
Raynaud's disease is a primary vasospastic process involving the small vessels of the upper extremity and

represents the most common form of upper extremity PAD. Upon exposure to cold or stress, the hand and fingers develop characteristic, sequential tricolored changes in appearance: initially the affected digits blanch to a very pale white color (*Figure 5*); then the color becomes dusky blue; and with rewarming and compensatory capillary vasodilatation, the color becomes red. The diagnosis may be confirmed with cold water immersion testing, where the color changes may be observed and the hand is slow to warm. Plethysmography may also demonstrate the development of peaked velocities during periods of vasospasm in the affected digits.

Treatment of Raynaud's includes preventive strategies such as avoiding cold, wearing gloves, and reducing stress. Calcium-channel blockers and alpha adrenergic blocking agents may be helpful to reduce vasospasm. Raynaud's syndrome—a secondary phenomenon—may occur in response to local conditions, such as TOS or local trauma, as well as with systemic disorders, such as autoinflammatory diseases (systemic lupus erythematosus, scleroderma, rheumatoid arthritis), or as a side effect from certain medications or drugs (beta-blockers, ergotamine-containing medications, illicit substances).[29]

Reflex sympathetic dystrophy—or complex regional pain syndrome (CRPS)—may involve a complex interplay between the sympathetic nervous system and the

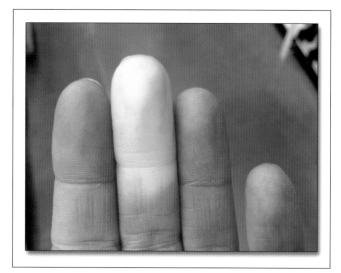

Figure 5

Photograph of the Left Hand in a Patient With Raynaud's Disease

Note the marked pallor of the distal third digit, due to microvascular spasm characteristic of Raynaud's Disease.

Image provided courtesy of Michael R. Jaff, DO, Massachusetts General Hospital, Boston, MA.

microcirculation of the distal portion of the affected limb. While specific mechanisms remain unclear, neurogenic inflammation and inhibition of local sympathetic tone during the acute phase of CRPS promote regional vasodilatation. Subsequently, the local rise in sympathetic tone causes vasoconstriction during the chronic phase of the disease. The associated skin warming during the acute phase and vasoconstriction with cooling in the chronic phase are classic stigmata of CRPS.[30]

Key Point

- In select cases, endovascular approaches may result in similar outcomes with fewer complications compared with surgical strategies for revascularization of patients with critical hypoperfusion due to upper extremity PAD. An individualized approach is required.

Conclusion

Upper extremity PAD is relatively uncommon and highly variable in its manifestations. Unlike lower extremity PAD, which is primarily caused by the development of atherosclerotic arterial narrowing, upper extremity PAD may occur in a variety of disease states affecting large and/or small arteries. Treatment and prevention require elucidation of the cause and understanding of its natural history.

References

1. Coletti A, Rajagopalan S. Approach to the patient with upper extremity arterial disease. In: Rajagopalan S, Mukherjee D, Mohler E, eds. Manual of Vascular Diseases. Philadelphia: Lippincott Williams & Wilkins; 2004:215-26.

2. Bartelink ML, Wollersheim H, Leesmans E, de Boo T, Thien T. A standardized finger cooling test for Raynaud's phenomenon: diagnostic value and sex differences. Eur Heart J 1993;14:614-22.

3. Aboyans V, Criqui MH, McDermott MM, et al. The vital prognosis of subclavian stenosis. J Am Coll Cardiol 2007;49:1540-5.

4. Weinberg I, Gona P, O'Donnell CJ, Jaff MR, Murabito JM. The systolic blood pressure difference between arms and cardiovascular disease in the Framingham Heart Study. Am J Med 2014;127:209-15.

5. Law MM, Colburn MD, Moore WS, Quiñones-Baldrich WJ, Machleder HI, Gelabert HA. Carotid-subclavian bypass for brachiocephalic occlusive disease. Choice of conduit and long-term follow-up. Stroke 1995;26:1565-71.

6. AbuRahma AF, Robinson PA, Jennings TG. Carotid-subclavian bypass grafting with polytetrafluoroethylene grafts for symptomatic subclavian artery stenosis or occlusion: a 20-year experience. J Vasc Surg 2000;32:411-8; discussion 418-9.

7. Patel SN, White CJ, Collins TJ, et al. Catheter-based treatment of the subclavian and innominate arteries. Catheter Cardiovasc Interv 2008;71:963-8.

8. Rogers JH, Calhoun RF 2nd. Diagnosis and management of subclavian artery stenosis prior to coronary artery bypass grafting in the current era. J Card Surg 2007;22:20-5.

9. Potter BJ, Pinto DS. Subclavian steal syndrome. Circulation 2014;129:2320-3.

10. Hadjipetrou P, Cox S, Piemonte T, Eisenhauer A. Percutaneous revascularization of atherosclerotic obstruction of aortic arch vessels. J Am Coll Cardiol 1999;33:1238-45.

11. Liu NH, LaBree LD, Feldon SE, Rao NA. The epidemiology of giant cell arteritis: a 12-year retrospective study. Ophthalmology 2001;108:1145-9.

12. Cid MC, Prieto-González S, Arguis P, et al. The spectrum of vascular involvement in giant-cell arteritis: clinical consequences of detrimental vascular remodelling at different sites. APMIS Suppl 2009:10-20.

13. Hayreh SS, Podhajsky PA, Raman R, Zimmerman B. Giant cell arteritis: validity and reliability of various diagnostic criteria. Am J Ophthalmol 1997;123:285-96.

14. Liozon E, Roblot P, Paire D, et al. Anticardiolipin antibody levels predict flares and relapses in patients with giant-cell (temporal) arteritis. A longitudinal study of 58 biopsy-proven cases. Rheumatology (Oxford) 2000;39:1089-94.

15. Kerr GS, Hallahan CW, Giordano J, et al. Takayasu arteritis. Ann Intern Med 1994;120:919-29.

16. Subramanyan R, Joy J, Balakrishnan KG. Natural history of aortoarteritis (Takayasu's disease). Circulation 1989;80:429-37.

17. Ishikawa K. Natural history and classification of occlusive thromboaortopathy (Takayasu's disease). Circulation 1978;57:27-35.

18. Min PK, Park S, Jung JH, et al. Endovascular therapy combined with immunosuppressive treatment for occlusive arterial disease in patients with Takayasu's arteritis. J Endovasc Ther 2005;12:28-34.

19. Ohta T, Ishioashi H, Hosaka M, Sugimoto I. Clinical and social consequences of Buerger disease. J Vasc Surg 2004;39:176-80.

20. Watson LA, Pizzari T, Balster S. Thoracic outlet syndrome part 1: clinical manifestations, differentiation and treatment pathways. Man Ther 2009;14:586-95.

21. Mackinnon SE, Novak CB. Evaluation of the patient with thoracic outlet syndrome. Semin Thorac Cardiovasc Surg 1996;8:190-200.

22. Marine L, Valdes F, Mertens R, Kramer A, Bergoeing M, Urbina J. Arterial thoracic outlet syndrome: a 32-year experience. Ann Vasc Surg 2013;27:1007-13.

23. Wagener JF, Rao SV. A comparison of radial and femoral access for cardiac catheterization. Trends Cardiovasc Med 2015;25:707-13.

24. Feldman DN, Swaminathan RV, Kaltenbach LA, et al. Adoption of radial access and comparison of outcomes to femoral access in percutaneous coronary intervention: an updated report from the national cardiovascular data registry (2007-2012). Circulation 2013;127:2295-306.

25. Kanei Y, Kwan T, Nakra NC, et al. Transradial cardiac catheterization: a review of access site complications. Catheter Cardiovasc Interv 2011;78:840-6.

26. Fisher RG, Whigham CJ, Trinh C. Diverticula of Kommerell and aberrant subclavian arteries complicated by aneurysms. Cardiovasc Intervent Radiol 2005;28:553-60.

27. Freed K, Low VH. The aberrant subclavian artery. AJR Am J Roentgenol 1997;168:481-4.

28. Stone WM, Ricotta JJ 2nd, Fowl RJ, Garg N, Bower TC, Money SR. Contemporary management of aberrant right subclavian arteries. Ann Vasc Surg 2011; 25:508-14.

29. Wigley FM. Clinical practice. Raynaud's Phenomenon. N Engl J Med 2002;347:1001-8.

30. Wasner G. Vasomotor disturbances in complex regional pain syndrome—a review. Pain Med 2010;11:1267-73.

Renal Artery Stenosis

Introduction

Renal artery stenosis (RAS), a common finding on abdominal imaging, has been implicated in the development of HTN and chronic kidney disease (CKD). While atherosclerosis is by far the most common etiology of renovascular HTN (~ 90% of cases), RAS may be a result of etiologies such as fibromuscular dysplasia (FMD), segmental arterial mediolysis, dissection, or arteritis. Treatment considerations must take into account the underlying cause. While medical therapy is the cornerstone of treatment, the indications for either surgical or transcatheter revascularization have been a matter of debate for nearly 2 decades.

Key Point

- Atherosclerosis is the most common cause of RAS.

Clinical Presentation

RAS is often diagnosed incidentally when imaging has been performed for unrelated reasons. Clinically, RAS should be suspected in the following scenarios:

- Resistant HTN, defined as the inability to achieve goal blood pressure of 140/90 mm Hg or lower despite the use of three antihypertensive medications at maximum tolerable doses used in appropriate combinations.[1]

- Poorly controlled HTN in a patient in whom blood pressure was previously easy to control.

- Early (before age 30) or late (after age 55) onset diastolic HTN. In early cases, etiologies other than atherosclerosis should be considered.

- Unexplained deterioration in renal function.

- Unexplained discrepancy in kidney size.

- Difficult to manage heart failure, especially if associated with unexplained episodes of "flash" pulmonary edema out of proportion to either left ventricular dysfunction or the burden of coronary artery disease.

HTN is associated with unilateral RAS (the 2 kidney, 1 clip model) through a failure of a feedback mechanism. The kidney ipsilateral to the stenosis responds by secreting renin, which promotes sodium retention and vasoconstriction via the renin-angiotensin-aldosterone pathway. This results in an increase in blood pressure. The contralateral kidney reacts by invoking a pressure natriuresis. Eventually, the contralateral kidney cannot compensate further and HTN develops in relation to angiotensin-II mediated systemic effects (*Figure 1*).[2] In patients with severe bilateral RAS, or severe unilateral RAS in a solitary kidney, HTN

Ido Weinberg, MD, MSc
Consultant Fees/Honoraria: VIVA Physicians.

Michael R. Jaff, DO, FACC
Consultant Fees/Honoraria: AOPA, Cardinal Health, Covidien, Micell Technologies, Vascular Therapies; Officer, Director, Trustee, or other Fiduciary Role: VIVA Physicians; Other – Non compensated advisor: Abbott Vascular, Boston Scientific, Cordis, IC Sciences, Medtronic Vascular; Other – Chair, Data Safety and Monitoring Board: Novello; Ownership Interest/Partnership/ Principal: Jana Care, MC10, Northwind Pharmaceuticals, PQ Bypass, Primacea, Sano V, Valiant Medical.

Learner Objectives

Upon completion of this module, the reader will be able to:

1. Identify patients with hypertension (HTN) who should be screened for renal artery stenosis (RAS).
2. Evaluate appropriate imaging options to identify renal artery stenosis.
3. Recognize the differences between atherosclerotic and nonatherosclerotic causes of RAS.
4. Select appropriate medical therapy for patients with RAS to reduce blood pressure, preserve renal function, and decrease cardiovascular events.
5. Incorporate recommendations for renal artery revascularization in appropriate patients.

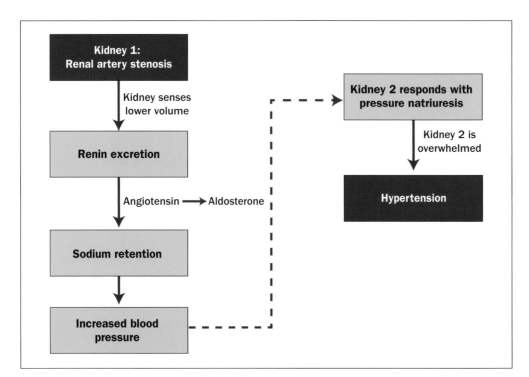

Figure 1
Mechanism of Renovascular Hypertension

is heavily dependent on the associated volume expansion as a result of impaired sodium and water excretion.

Renal failure in patients with atherosclerotic RAS, on the other hand, has several potential explanations. It may result from long-standing systemic HTN, renal ischemia, recurrent atheromatous embolization, or from contrast nephropathy following imaging studies.[3]

The natural history of atherosclerotic RAS is incompletely understood. While atherosclerotic RAS is found more often in patients with end-stage renal disease (ESRD) than in the general population,[4] there is not a linear relationship between the degree of atherosclerotic RAS and HTN or CKD.[5] In a retrospective analysis of 96 patients with incidentally noted atherosclerotic RAS, the temporal change in serum creatinine or risk of death did not correlate with the baseline degree of stenosis.[6] Nonetheless, atherosclerotic RAS may be progressive, leading to more severe stenosis, occlusion of the renal artery, and renal atrophy.[7,8] In a retrospective analysis of serial renal angiographic studies in 85 patients with atherosclerotic RAS, 44% demonstrated progression of stenosis severity over 52 months, with 16% progressing to renal artery occlusion. Baseline stenosis >75% predicted both progression of disease and progression to occlusion.[8] In a prospective study, 44% of patients showed progressive renal artery narrowing over time. The risk of renal atrophy in this study was higher in patients with RAS at baseline compared with patients in whom no RAS was present.[7] In a small trial, 32 patients with incidentally discovered atherosclerotic RAS were compared with 139 patients without RAS. After 6.3 years of follow-up, patients with atherosclerotic RAS were more likely to develop HTN, and in those with HTN, more medications were required for

blood pressure control. Of note, there was no progression of renal dysfunction nor an increase in mortality risk among patients with atherosclerotic RAS.[9] Lack of progressive renal dysfunction in patients treated medically was also seen in the CORAL (Cardiovascular Outcomes in Renal Atherosclerotic Lesions) trial.[10]

The consequences of RAS as a result of FMD are different. While these patients may have loss of renal parenchyma, they usually do not present with CKD, but rather with HTN. Progression to renal failure is uncommon.[11]

Key Point

- The diagnosis of clinically significant RAS should be considered in patients with early onset (age <30) or late-onset (age >55) HTN, previously well-controlled HTN that has escaped, and recurrent heart failure exacerbations or "flash" pulmonary edema out of proportion to left ventricular systolic dysfunction, or the burden of coronary artery disease.

Epidemiology

Atherosclerotic RAS affected 6.8% of patients in the Cardiovascular Health Study, a population-based study of elderly subjects.[12] It is even more prevalent in at-risk populations, including patients with poorly controlled HTN[13] or atherosclerosis in other vascular beds,[14] most specifically among patients with coronary artery disease (18-20%)[15] or peripheral artery disease, where it has been found in up to 59% of patients.[16] The true prevalence of FMD is less clear. While likely under-reported, it probably

Condition	Imaging Clue	Clinical Characteristics
Atherosclerosis	Ostial involvement; often contiguous with aortic atherosclerotic disease; atherosclerosis in other vascular beds (e.g., coronary, carotid, iliofemoral, infra-inguinal)	Prevalence increases with age; incidentally noted; may be associated with new-onset or difficult to control hypertension; may be associated with deteriorating renal function
Fibromuscular Dysplasia	The most common type has a "beaded" appearance; typically involves the distal portion of the artery; may be associated with aneurysm formation or dissection; other vascular beds (e.g., carotid, coronary) may be involved	Most commonly noted in young or middle-aged women; usually not associated with impaired renal function
Large Artery Vasculitis	Peri-arterial enhancement on MRA or CTA	Often associated with markers of systemic inflammation
Segmental Arterial Mediolysis	Long, smooth segments of stenosis	Unknown; may present locally or involve multiple arteries ("catastrophic" form)

Table 1
Causes of Renal Artery Stenosis

CTA = computed tomography angiography; MRA = magnetic resonance angiography.

accounts for <10% of RAS and only 5-10% of cases renovascular HTN.[17]

Differential Diagnosis

The recognized causes of RAS and some of their distinguishing characteristics are listed in *Table 1*.

Key Points

- Atherosclerotic renal artery disease typically affects the ostium and proximal part of the artery, from direct extension of disease within the aorta.

- FMD, the second most common cause of renal artery stenosis, most often affects young or middle-aged women and affects the mid-to-distal portion of the renal artery. The most common form of FMD is beaded in its angiographic appearance.

Diagnosis

RAS is often diagnosed incidentally. Nonetheless, caution should be exercised in drawing conclusions regarding renal artery anatomy from nondedicated imaging, as proper technique is important in making a correct diagnosis. The diagnosis of RAS can be established with renal artery duplex ultrasound (RADUS), computed tomography angiography (CTA), magnetic resonance angiography (MRA), or contrast angiography. A stepwise use of these modalities is advised (*Figure 2*).[18] *Table 2*

outlines imaging modality characteristics as well as their relative advantages and disadvantages.

Captopril renal scintigraphy, while having a sound theoretical basis, does not have acceptable sensitivity for the diagnosis of RAS, and has not been consistently shown to predict outcome.[19] It is rarely used in current practice and is not routinely recommended.

RADUS is a reasonable, noninvasive option for confirming the diagnosis and for surveillance of RAS. It is accurate, inexpensive, painless, and does not involve ionizing radiation or contrast agents (*Figure 3*). Ultrasound criteria for the diagnosis of RAS depend on peak systolic velocities (PSV) within the renal artery, as well as the ratio of the PSV at the level of the renal artery origin and the PSV as measured in the aorta at the level of the superior mesenteric artery. This ratio is known as the renal/aortic ratio (RAR). A RAR >3.5 is usually indicative of stenosis; however, criteria vary between centers. Importantly, RADUS does not offer a specific percent of stenosis, but rather provides categorization of RAS into broad ranges of stenosis (e.g., 0-59%, 60-99%, and occluded), much like carotid duplex scanning. The utility of RADUS was demonstrated in a prospective series comparing 102 RADUS exams to contrast angiography. The sensitivity of RADUS was 98%, specificity 99%, positive predictive value 99%, and negative predictive value 97%.[20] Small series also have shown RADUS to be useful for the diagnosis and surveillance of renal artery FMD. Ultrasound may identify the typical beaded appearance of the most common variant of FMD (medial fibroplasia variant), and elevated PSV measurements may

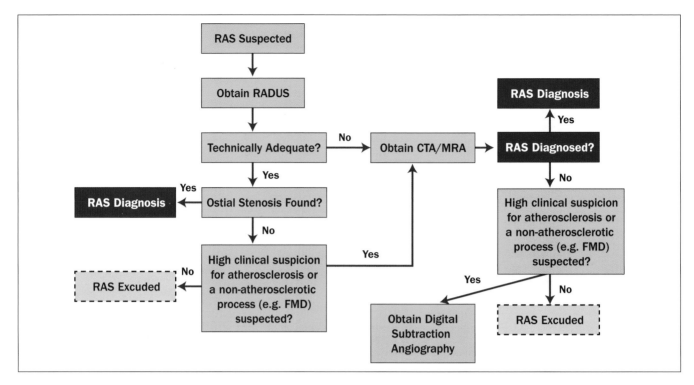

Figure 2

Algorithmic Approach to the Diagnosis of Renal Artery Stenosis

CTA = computed tomography angiography; FMD = fibromuscular dysplasia; MRA = magnetic resonance angiography; RAS = renal artery stenosis; RADUS = renal artery duplex ultrasound.

	Advantages	Disadvantages	When Should This Imaging Be Used?
RADUS	Accurate, inexpensive, painless, does not involve ionizing radiation or contrast agents	Requires technical expertise, less accurate in visualizing accessory arteries, limited extra-renal anatomical information, patient characteristics may hinder image acquisition	Preliminary screening, surveillance of known RAS, post-procedural surveillance
CTA	Offers anatomic definition of main and accessory renal arteries, visualization of structures beyond the renal artery, ability to identify and assess the progression of other pathologies within the renal artery (e.g., aneurysms)	Ionizing radiation, exposure to contrast, poor quality in calcified lesions, less accurate in distal portions of the renal artery	Commonly used to plan procedures, confirmation of FMD, surveillance of non- stenotic lesions (e.g., aneurysms)
MRA		Contrast exposure, not compatible with most ICDs or PPMs, unable to visualize stented arteries, poor quality in distal portions of the renal artery	
Angiography	"Gold standard" in evaluating degree of RAS	Invasive procedure, limited extra-arterial anatomical information, involves ionizing radiation and contrast	Confirmation of ambiguous findings on other imaging studies, when a procedure is probable

Table 2

Comparison of Imaging Modalities for Diagnosis and/or Surveillance of RAS

CTA = computed tomography angiography; FMD = fibromuscular dysplasia, ICDs = implantable cardioverter-defibrillators; MRA = magnetic resonance angiography; PPMs = permanent pacemakers; RADUS = renal artery duplex ultrasonography; RAS = renal artery stenosis.

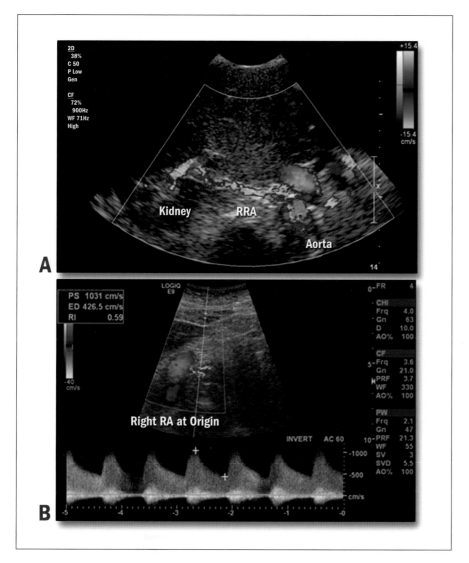

Figure 3
Renal Artery Duplex Ultrasonography

Panel A: Color-flow duplex ultrasound images taken from the right flank approach showing the aorta, right renal artery (RRA), and the kidney. There is turbulence in the RRA; however, no statement can be made about degree of narrowing in the absence of Doppler-derived flow velocity measurements.

Panel B: Pulse-wave Doppler images taken from the transabdominal approach showing elevated peak systolic and end-diastolic velocities at the origin of the right renal artery (RA) indicating stenosis of 60-99%.

suggest mid or distal artery involvement.[21] Nonetheless, RADUS does have limitations. It requires technical competence, including the need for specially trained technologists and skilled physicians to perform and interpret the results. Other limitations include difficulty visualizing the renal arteries with overlying bowel gas or morbid obesity, the challenge of identifying polar (accessory) renal arteries, and the delineation of distal renal artery disease.[22]

Both CTA and MRA are useful in providing information about renal artery anatomy (*Figure 4*). They should be used when RADUS is not technically adequate or when RADUS is normal, yet a high clinical suspicion for RAS or for another structural abnormality in the renal arteries (e.g., FMD) remains. Advantages include superior spatial resolution, ability to provide three-dimensional reconstruction of the anatomy, rapid identification of accessory (polar) renal arteries, visualization of the abdominal aorta and kidneys, and the ability to identify and assess other vascular pathologies, including aneurysms, which may complicate both atherosclerosis and FMD.[21] A meta-analysis found high discriminatory value for both CTA and MRA in the diagnosis of atherosclerotic RAS. Areas under the receiver-operating characteristic curves were 0.99 for CTA, 0.99 for gadolinium-enhanced MRA, and 0.97 for nongadolinium-enhanced MRA.[23] Nonetheless, CTA and MRA are not without limitations. CTA is challenged by the presence of arterial calcifications, potentially obscuring the arterial lumen. MRA has a tendency to overestimate the severity of arterial stenoses, and cannot visualize arterial segments within metallic stents because of signal dropout. CTA and MRA are also limited in their ability to assess distal RAS, which may hinder their ability to detect FMD.[24] CTA mandates the use of iodinated contrast and ionizing radiation, therefore making it an unattractive method for serial surveillance of RAS. Many patients cannot undergo MRA because of claustrophobia or indwelling metallic implants, including pacemakers, defibrillators, and certain renal artery stents. Gadolinium-based contrast agents used in MRA acquisition are associated with a risk of nephrogenic systemic sclerosis in patients with CKD. While techniques exist to acquire MRA-based images of the renal arteries without contrast, these are not widely available; many experts believe that gadolinium is required to accurately evaluate renal artery anatomy.

Catheter-based angiography is still considered the "gold standard" for the diagnosis of RAS. Other than its accuracy, advantages of angiography include the ability to acquire multiple images at various angles and to reliably identify accessory vessels and other anatomical variants. Invasive angiography should be performed only if other studies fail to show RAS and a high clinical suspicion remains.

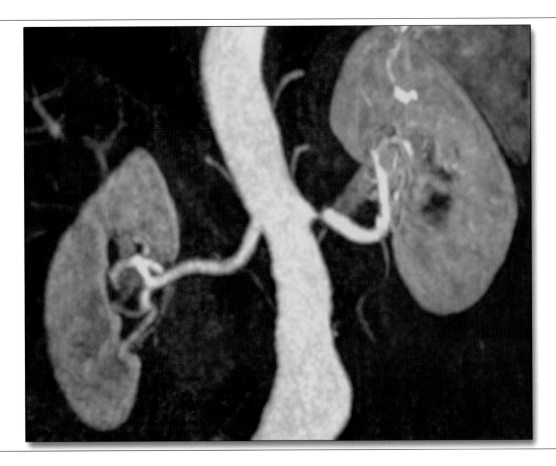

Figure 4

Computed Tomography Angiography Reconstruction Showing Proximal Left Renal Artery Stenosis

Angiography is considered the most accurate approach for diagnosis of FMD as it can reliably evaluate the distal portions of the renal artery.[21] Intravascular ultrasound (IVUS) and/or translesional pressure measurements are often needed to evaluate the hemodynamic significance of a stenosis in renal artery FMD, as it is incorrect to assess this visually.[11,25] Limitations of angiography include its invasive nature, exposure to ionizing radiation, and the need for contrast. Also, angiography does not provide information about structures in and around the kidneys.

> **Key Point**
>
> - Duplex ultrasonography should be used as the first imaging modality to screen for RAS. If further imaging is needed, CTA or MRA may be useful. The gold standard for diagnosis is invasive angiography, but it should be used judiciously.

Treatment

Medical Therapy

Medical and lifestyle therapies directed at atherosclerotic cardiovascular disease risk factors are the mainstay of treatment of atherosclerotic RAS. Patients with atherosclerotic RAS, like those with peripheral artery disease, incur excess morbidity and mortality from heart disease (i.e., myocardial infarction) and stroke. In addition to blood pressure management, therapies include lipid-lowering interventions (with statins whenever possible), tobacco cessation, glycemic control, antiplatelet agents (e.g., aspirin), diet, and exercise.[26] The effect of statins on mortality and renal outcomes was examined in a retrospective case-control study of 104 patients with atherosclerotic RAS who were followed for up to 134 months.[27] Patients treated with statins were less likely to die or double their serum creatinine levels, and fewer were likely to progress to ESRD. Presently, blood pressure reduction should target the goals recommended by the panel members appointed to the Eighth Joint National Committee, namely, <140/90 mm Hg, or <130/80 mm Hg in patients with diabetes or CKD.[28] These targets are subject to change with incorporation of the results of recent blood pressure reduction trials. Angiotensin-converting enzyme inhibitors (ACEIs) are preferred in patients with unilateral atherosclerotic RAS, as recommended by current practice guidelines.[16] Angiotensin-receptor blockers (ARBs) are recommended for ACEI-intolerant patients. Patients with bilateral RAS may develop worsening renal insufficiency

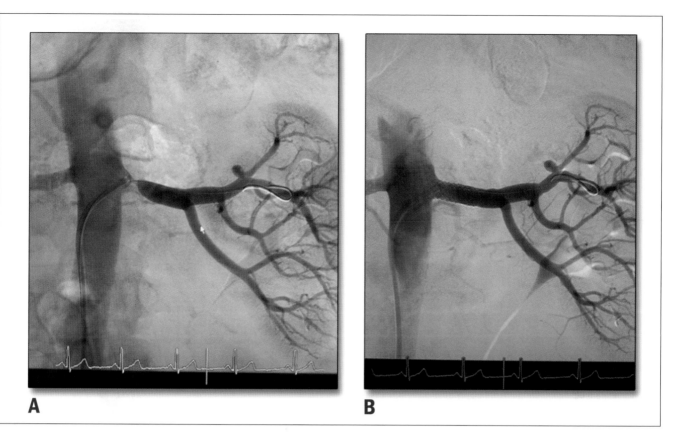

Figure 5

Digital Subtraction Angiography of the Left Renal Artery

Panel A: Digital subtraction angiography showing ostial left renal artery stenosis.

Panel B: Digital subtraction angiography showing resolution of the stenosis with a renal artery stent in place.

or hyperkalemia after exposure to ACEIs or ARBs. A retrospective evaluation of 190 patients treated with either revascularization or medical therapy showed a clear survival benefit for patients treated with ACEIs over a mean follow-up of 54 months, independent of revascularization status.[29] Beta-blockers and calcium channel blockers also can be used to treat renovascular HTN.[16]

Medical treatment in FMD-related RAS has not been extensively studied. It is customary to treat patients with FMD with an antiplatelet agent and anti-HTN medications.[21,30]

Endovascular Treatment

Endovascular interventions have been utilized for the treatment of RAS for more than 4 decades (*Figure 5*).[31]

Indications

The efficacy of endovascular therapy for atherosclerotic RAS has proven to be more limited than previously thought. Although a meta-analysis of multicenter Food and Drug Administration-approved investigational device exemption studies of renal artery stent revascularization in hypertensive patients with RAS showed a significant reduction in blood pressure,[32] the results of randomized controlled trials have been less convincing. Current practice

guidelines regarding the use of endovascular therapy are appropriately conservative. Endovascular therapy is indicated (Class I) in patients with severe RAS and unexplained heart failure or sudden, unexplained (flash) pulmonary edema. Endovascular therapy is reasonable (Class IIa) in patients with hemodynamically significant RAS and accelerated, resistant, or malignant HTN; HTN with an unexplained unilateral small kidney; HTN with intolerance to medications; progressive CKD with bilateral disease or disease affecting a solitary kidney; or unstable angina. The usefulness of endovascular therapy is uncertain (Class IIb) for treatment of asymptomatic bilateral RAS or RAS in a solitary viable kidney, asymptomatic unilateral RAS in a viable kidney, and unilateral RAS with CKD.[33] Other subgroups of patients may benefit from endovascular therapy, but decision making must be individualized.

Patients with FMD also may be treated with catheter-based intervention (*Figure 6*), but the indications for catheter-based treatment have not been well validated. They would include intervention with the intent to cure new-onset HTN or HTN with intolerance to medications. Surprisingly, a recent meta-analysis reporting the results of 47 trials of percutaneous transluminal renal angioplasty (PTRA)

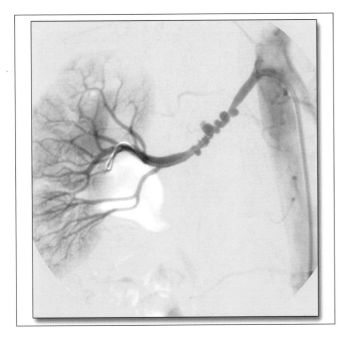

Figure 6

Selective Digital Subtraction Angiography of the Right Renal Artery Revealing the Characteristic Beaded Appearance of the Medial Fibroplasia Subtype of Fibromuscular Dysplasia

in FMD patients with HTN noted that the blood pressure response rate was only 47.5%.[34]

Technique

As the mechanism underlying atherosclerotic RAS is often bulky atheromatous aorto-renal plaque, PTRA does not provide durable patency. Endovascular renal artery stent revascularization (RASR), on the other hand, offers an acute procedural success rate of up to 98%.[35] Multiple comparisons have shown superiority of RASR over PTRA in renal artery revascularization. For example, in a prospective randomized study, procedural success rate was reported to be 57% in 40 patients who underwent PTRA and 88% in 41 patients who underwent RASR.[36] In the STAR (Stenting in Renal Dysfunction Caused by Atherosclerotic Renal Artery Stenosis) trial, only 2 out of 62 (3.2%) patients treated with renal artery stents experienced restenosis at 2 years follow-up.[37] In the HERCULES trial, a balloon expandable stent (Abbott Vascular, Santa Clara, CA) was used to treat 241 lesions; restenosis developed in 10.5% of patients at 9 months.[38]

As opposed to atherosclerotic RAS, FMD lesions often respond favorably to PTRA alone. Restenosis in patients with FMD is usually a result of inadequate balloon inflation during the first intervention and is classically managed with repeat PTRA.[21,39] Stents are used only in resistant cases, to manage complications or to exclude an aneurysm. With FMD, IVUS is often used to help target culprit lesions, as multiple intra-arterial bands may be present in a single artery.[11]

Key Points

- Patients with atherosclerotic RAS should be treated with aggressive risk-factor reduction strategies and antihypertensive medications.

- Endovascular renal artery revascularization is indicated (Class I) in patients with severe RAS and unexplained heart failure or sudden, unexplained (flash) pulmonary edema.

- Endovascular therapy is reasonable (Class IIa) in patients with hemodynamically significant RAS and accelerated, resistant, or malignant HTN; HTN with an unexplained unilateral small kidney; HTN with intolerance to medications; progressive CKD with bilateral disease or disease affecting a solitary kidney; or unstable angina.

- The usefulness of endovascular therapy is uncertain (Class IIb) for treatment of asymptomatic bilateral RAS or RAS in a solitary viable kidney, asymptomatic unilateral RAS in a viable kidney, and unilateral RAS with CKD.

Outcomes

Despite the inherent logic of revascularization to improve renal blood flow and the promising results of observational studies, several prospective randomized trials have failed to show convincing superiority of interventional therapy over medical treatment for management of atherosclerotic RAS. Although many trials have been flawed, the bulk of the data points are against benefit for procedural intervention in most atherosclerotic RAS patients. An inventory of the major trials is presented in *Table 3*. While an in-depth discussion of each is beyond the scope of this chapter, the largest and most recent study to date comparing intervention with medical therapy in patients with atherosclerotic RAS, the CORAL (Cardiovascular Outcomes in Renal Atherosclerotic Lesions) trial, deserves mention.[10] This study randomized 947 patients who had at least 60% stenosis of their renal artery and had either systolic HTN not well managed on at least two medications or CKD. Only patients for whom equipoise existed regarding the potential benefit of a revascularization procedure were randomized. At a median follow-up of 43 months, no benefit in either renal function or blood pressure control was found for intervention compared with medical therapy alone. While critics would claim that 60% lesion severity is a relatively modest threshold, none of the subgroup analyses showed benefit with intervention, including among patients with >80% stenoses. The lack of demonstrated benefit could have been related to the trial having been underpowered, but also suggests that any benefit associated with interventions was likely small.[40]

	DRASTIC[1]	STAR[2]	ASTRAL[3]	CORAL[4]
Year of publication	2000	2009	2009	2014
Primary endpoint	Blood pressure reduction	Renal function	Renal function	Major cardiovascular or renal event
Inclusion	HTN, RAS >50%, Cr<2.3 mg/dl	Cl_{Cr} <80ml/min, RAS>50%	RAS*	Originally RAS and HTN, revised to include RAS and GFR<60 ml/min/1.73m^2
Number of patients (control/intervention)	56/50	64/74	403/403	472/459
Mean follow-up (months)	12	33.6	24	43
% stent in intervention arm	3.4	98.4	95	94.6
% of patients experiencing any complication	28.3	15.7	29	5.2
Inclusion of patients who were later found not to have significant renal artery stenosis	+	+	+	+/-¥
Outcome in revascularization arm	Improved BP control, fewer medications needed to control HTN	No improvement in renal function compared to medical arm	Trend toward slower renal function decline, fewer medications needed to control HTN	No difference between groups in the composite primary endpoint, individual components of the endpoint, and subgroup analyses. 2.3 mm Hg difference in systolic BP favoring the stent group.

Table 3

Comparison of Renal Artery Intervention Trials

* Atherosclerotic RAS was suspected if there was HTN or unexplained renal dysfunction.

¥ The threshold definition of significant atherosclerotic RAS was lowered during the study.

BP = blood pressure; Cl_{Cr} = creatinine clearance; Cr = creatinine; GFR = glomerular filtration rate; HTN = hypertension; RAS = renal artery stenosis.

References:

1. van Jaarsveld BC, Krijnen P, Pieterman H, et al. The effect of balloon angioplasty on hypertension in atherosclerotic renal-artery stenosis. Dutch Renal Artery Stenosis Intervention Cooperative Study Group. N Engl J Med 2000;342:1007-14.

2. Bax L, Woittiez AJ, Kouwenberg HJ, et al. Stent placement in patients with atherosclerotic renal artery stenosis and impaired renal function: a randomized trial. Ann Intern Med 2009;150:840-8.

3. ASTRAL Investigators, Wheatley K, Ives N, et al. Revascularization versus medical therapy for renal-artery stenosis. N Engl J Med 2009;361:1953-62.

4. Cooper CJ, Murphy TP, Cutlip DE, et al., on behalf of the CORAL Investigators. Stenting and medical therapy for atherosclerotic renal-artery stenosis. N Engl J Med 2014;370:13-22.

Complications

Endovascular RAS treatment is not devoid of risk. Complications include local access site and systemic complications including hematoma, retroperitoneal hemorrhage, pseudoaneurysm, deterioration in renal function, renal artery dissection, renal artery occlusion, renal artery perforation, and death.[37,41-45] Although reported complication rates of up to 28.3% have been described,[43] serious adverse effects are usually far less common. For example, the serious adverse event rate at 30 days in HERCULES was only 1.5%.[38] In the CORAL trial, angiographic complications were noted in approximately 5% of patients.[10] Worsening renal function is of particular importance in RAS patients and, in the context of intervention, may be a result of atheromatous embolization and/or contrast-related nephrotoxicity. Athero-emboli have been demonstrated in >50% of cases with distal embolic protection devices.[46]

Surveillance

Patients with RAS who are being treated medically should be monitored for medication side-effects, quality of blood pressure control, deterioration in renal function, or progressive renal atrophy. RADUS remains the most useful tool for routine surveillance of both native and stented renal arteries. There are no high-quality data to guide surveillance protocols; however, appropriate use criteria have been defined.[47] An acceptable protocol for surveillance of atherosclerotic RAS is based on the etiology, clinical scenario, and anatomic findings. For native arteries, after a preliminary diagnosis, a repeat examination usually can be considered at 6 months to screen for early progression. Thereafter, patients usually are enrolled in an annual surveillance program. Factors that may prompt more frequent testing include deterioration in blood pressure control, symptoms of cardio-renal syndrome, progressive renal dysfunction, or renal atrophy. As with native arteries, surveillance following RASR should incorporate both clinical and imaging data. Again, there are few data to guide the development of surveillance protocols. A single-center, retrospective analysis of 1,150 RASR procedures performed over 10 years found an overall need for reintervention in 11%, most within the first 2 years and most often in patients presenting with recurrent HTN.[48] The criteria for in-stent restenosis have not been rigorously defined. Suggested criteria for in-stent restenosis >60% include a PSV ≥296 cm/sec with poststenotic turbulence and/or a RAR of ≥4.4. A PSV <241 cm/sec accurately excludes significant restenosis.[49] Based on these data and per convention, patients usually are followed by RADUS soon after stent placement, at 6 and 12 months, and annually thereafter.

Surveillance of FMD-related RAS should take into account the potential systemic nature of this condition. FMD most commonly affects the renal and extracranial carotid arteries.[50] By convention, postprocedural surveillance for FMD is recommended soon after the procedure, at 6 and 12 months, and yearly thereafter.[11,21] Importantly, restenosis is not always an adequate indication to prompt re-intervention, as there may be a poor correlation between imaging and clinical presentations.[51]

Periprocedural medical therapy to improve short- and long-term outcomes after endovascular intervention also has not been rigorously assessed.[52] It is customary to treat patients with an antiplatelet agent such as aspirin or clopidogrel indefinitely after intervention. Dual antiplatelet therapy also has been used.

Surgery

Surgical repair for isolated RAS has a very limited role. Surgery remains a valid option for selected patients with renal artery aneurysms not amenable to endovascular treatment and for patients with extensive atherosclerotic/aneurysmal disease affecting the contiguous aorta.

Future Directions

As RASR has repeatedly failed to show benefit in both the general atherosclerotic RAS population and many FMD patients with RAS, further research is needed to identify patients prospectively for whom revascularization would be helpful. More information about the natural history and treatment of FMD is expected to become available from a US registry over the coming years.[50]

References

1. Textor SC. Current approaches to renovascular hypertension. Med Clin North Am 2009;93:717-32.

2. Garovic VD, Textor SC. Renovascular hypertension and ischemic nephropathy. Circulation 2005;112:1362-74.

3. Manske CL, Sprafka JM, Strony JT, Wang Y. Contrast nephropathy in azotemic diabetic patients undergoing coronary angiography. Am J Med 1990;89:615-20.

4. Guzman RP, Zierler RE, Isaacson JA, Bergelin RO, Strandness DE Jr. Renal atrophy and arterial stenosis. A prospective study with duplex ultrasound. Hypertension 1994;23:346-50.

5. Chrysochou C, Kalra PA. Epidemiology and natural history of atherosclerotic renovascular disease. Prog Cardiovasc Dis 2009;52:184-95.

6. Iglesias JI, Hamburger RJ, Feldman L, Kaufman JS. The natural history of incidental renal artery stenosis in patients with aortoiliac vascular disease. Am J Med 2000;109:642-7.

7. Caps MT, Zierler RE, Polissar NL, et al. Risk of atrophy in kidneys with atherosclerotic renal artery stenosis. Kidney Int 1998;53:735-42.

8. Schreiber MJ, Pohl MA, Novick AC. The natural history of atherosclerotic and fibrous renal artery disease. Urol Clin North Am 1984;11:383-92.

9. Williamson WK, Abou-Zamzam AM Jr, Moneta GL, et al. Prophylactic repair of renal artery stenosis is not justified in patients who require infrarenal aortic reconstruction. J Vasc Surg 1998;28:14-20.

10. Cooper CJ, Murphy TP, Cutlip DE, et al. Stenting and medical therapy for atherosclerotic renal-artery stenosis. N Engl J Med 2014;370:13-22.

11. Slovut DP, Olin JW. Fibromuscular dysplasia. N Engl J Med 2004;350:1862-71.

12. Hansen KJ, Edwards MS, Craven TE, et al. Prevalence of renovascular disease in the elderly: a population-based study. J Vasc Surg 2002;36:443-51.

13. Davis RP, Pearce JD, Craven TE, et al. Atherosclerotic renovascular disease among hypertensive adults. J Vasc Surg 2009;50:564-70.

14. Olin JW, Melia M, Young JR, Graor RA, Risius B. Prevalence of atherosclerotic renal artery stenosis in patients with atherosclerosis elsewhere. Am J Med 1990;88:46N-51N.

15. Rihal CS, Textor SC, Breen JF, et al. Incidental renal artery stenosis among a prospective cohort of hypertensive patients undergoing coronary angiography. Mayo Clin Proc 2002;77:309-16.

16. Hirsch AT, Haskal ZJ, Hertzer NR, et al. ACC/AHA 2005 guidelines for the management of patients with peripheral arterial disease (lower extremity, renal, mesenteric, and abdominal aortic): a collaborative report from the American Association

for Vascular Surgery/Society for Vascular Surgery, Society for Cardiovascular Angiography and Interventions, Society for Vascular Medicine and Biology, Society of Interventional Radiology, and the ACC/AHA Task Force on Practice Guidelines (Writing Committee to Develop Guidelines for the Management of Patients With Peripheral Arterial Disease). J Am Coll Cardiol. 2006;47::e1-e192.

17. Safian RD, Textor SC. Renal-artery stenosis. N Engl J Med 2001;344:431-42.

18. Dworkin LD, Cooper CJ. Clinical practice. Renal-artery stenosis. N Engl J Med 2009;361:1972-8.

19. Soulez G, Therasse E, Qanadi SD, et al. Prediction of clinical response after renal angioplasty: respective value of renal Doppler sonography and scintigraphy. AJR Am J Roentgenol 2003;181:1029-35.

20. Olin JW, Piedmonte MR, Young JR, DeAnna S, Grubb M, Childs MB. The utility of duplex ultrasound scanning of the renal arteries for diagnosing significant renal artery stenosis. Ann Intern Med 1995;122:833-8.

21. Olin JW, Sealove BA. Diagnosis, management, and future developments of fibromuscular dysplasia. J Vasc Surg 2011;53:826-36.

22. Das CJ, Neyaz Z, Thapa P, Sharma S, Vashist S Fibromuscular dysplasia of the renal arteries: a radiological review. Int Urol Nephrol 2007;39:233-8.

23. Vasbinder GB, Nelemans PJ, Kessels AG, Kroon AA, de Leeuw PW, van Engelshoven JM. Diagnostic tests for renal artery stenosis in patients suspected of having renovascular hypertension: a meta-analysis. Ann Intern Med 2001;135:401-11.

24. Tan KT, van Beek EJ, Brown PW, van Delden OM, Tijssen J, Ramsay LE. Magnetic resonance angiography for the diagnosis of renal artery stenosis: a meta-analysis. Clin Radiol 2002;57:617-24.

25. Gowda MS, Loeb AL, Crouse LJ, Kramer PH. Complementary roles of color-flow duplex imaging and intravascular ultrasound in the diagnosis of renal artery fibromuscular dysplasia: should renal arteriography serve as the "gold standard"? J Am Coll Cardiol 2003;41:1305-11.

26. Reich SB. Renal-artery stenosis. New Engl J Med 2001;345:221.

27. Silva VS, Martin LC, Franco RJ, et al. Pleiotropic effects of statins may improve outcomes in atherosclerotic renovascular disease. Am J Hypertens 2008;21:1163-8.

28. James PA, Oparil S, Carter BL, et al. 2014 evidence-based guideline for the management of high blood pressure in adults: report from the panel members appointed to the Eighth Joint National Committee (JNC 8). JAMA 2014;311:507-20.

29. Losito A, Errico R, Santirosi P, Lupattelli T, Scalera GB, Lupattelli L. Long-term follow-up of atherosclerotic renovascular disease. Beneficial effect of ACE inhibition. Nephrol Dial Transplant 2005;20:1604-9.

30. Weinberg I, Gu X, Giri J, et al. Anti-platelet and anti-hypertension medication use in patients with fibromuscular dysplasia: results from the United States Registry for Fibromuscular Dysplasia. Vasc Med 2015;20:447-53.

31. Ying CY, Tifft CP, Gavras H, Chobanian AV. Renal revascularization in the azotemic hypertensive patient resistant to therapy. N Engl J Med 1984;311:1070-5.

32. Weinberg I, Keyes MJ, Giri J, et al. Blood pressure response to renal artery stenting in 901 patients from five prospective multicenter FDA-approved trials. Catheter Cardiovasc Interv 2014;83:603-9.

33. Parikh SA, Shishehbor MH, Gray BH, White CJ, Jaff MR. SCAI expert consensus statement for renal artery stenting appropriate use. Catheter Cardiovasc Interv 2014;84:1163-71.

34. Trinquart L, Mounier-Vehier C, Sapoval M, Gagnon N, Plouin PF. Efficacy of revascularization for renal artery stenosis caused by fibromuscular dysplasia: a systematic review and meta-analysis. Hypertension 2010;56:525-32.

35. Simon JF. Stenting atherosclerotic renal arteries: time to be less aggressive. Cleve Clin J Med 2010;77:178-89.

36. van de Ven PJ, Kaatee R, Beutler JJ, et al. Arterial stenting and balloon angioplasty in ostial atherosclerotic renovascular disease: a randomised trial. Lancet 1999;353:282-6.

37. Bax L, Woittiez AJ, Kouwenberg HJ, et al. Stent placement in patients with atherosclerotic renal artery stenosis and impaired renal function: a randomized trial. Ann Intern Med 2009;150:840-8.

38. Jaff MR, Bates M, Sullivan T, et al., on behalf of the HERCULES Investigators. Significant reduction in systolic blood pressure following renal artery stenting in patients with uncontrolled hypertension: results from the HERCULES trial. Catheter Cardiovasc Interv 2012;80:343-50.

39. Sos TA, Pickering TG, Sniderman K, et al. Percutaneous transluminal renal angioplasty in renovascular hypertension due to atheroma or fibromuscular dysplasia. N Engl J Med 1983;309:274-9.

40. Bittl JA. Treatment of atherosclerotic renovascular disease. N Engl J Med 2014;370:78-9.

41. Plouin PF, Chatellier G, Darné B, Raynaud A. Blood pressure outcome of angioplasty in atherosclerotic renal artery stenosis: a randomized trial. Essai Multicentrique Medicaments vs Angioplastie (EMMA) Study Group. Hypertension 1998;31:823-9.

42. Webster J, Marshall F, Abdalla M, et al. Randomised comparison of percutaneous angioplasty vs continued medical therapy for hypertensive patients with atheromatous renal artery stenosis. Scottish and Newcastle Renal Artery Stenosis Collaborative Group. J Hum Hypertens 1998;12:329-35.

43. van Jaarsveld BC, Krijnen P, Pieterman H, et al. The effect of balloon angioplasty on hypertension in atherosclerotic renal-artery stenosis. Dutch Renal Artery Stenosis Intervention Cooperative Study Group. N Engl J Med 2000;342:1007-14.

44. Rocha-Singh K, Jaff MR, Rosenfield K, on behalf of the ASPIRE-2 Trial Investigators. Evaluation of the safety and effectiveness of renal artery stenting after unsuccessful balloon angioplasty: the ASPIRE-2 study. J Am Coll Cardiol 2005;46:776-83.

45. ASTRAL Investigators, Wheatley K, Ives N, Gray R, et al. Revascularization versus medical therapy for renal-artery stenosis. N Engl J Med 2009;361:1953-62.

46. Henry M, Henry I, Klonaris C, et al. Renal angioplasty and stenting under protection: the way for the future? Catheter Cardiovasc Interv 2003;60:299-312.

47. Mohler ER 3rd, Gornik HL, Gerhard-Herman M, Misra S, Olin JW, Zierler E. ACCF/ACR/AIUM/ASE/ASN/ICAVL/SCAI/SCCT/SIR/SVM/SVS 2012 appropriate use criteria for peripheral vascular ultrasound and physiological testing part I: arterial ultrasound and physiological testing. J Vasc Surg 2012;56:e17-51.

48. Stone PA, Campbell JE, Aburahma AF, et al. Ten-year experience with renal artery in-stent stenosis. J Vasc Surg 2011;53:1026-31.

49. Del Conde I, Galin ID, Trost B, et al. Renal artery duplex ultrasound criteria for the detection of significant in-stent restenosis. Catheter Cardiovasc Interv 2014;83:612-8.

50. Olin JW, Froehlich J, Gu X, et al. The United States Registry for Fibromuscular Dysplasia: results in the first 447 patients. Circulation 2012;125:3182-90.

51. Birrer M, Do DD, Mahler F, Triller J, Baumgartner I. Treatment of renal artery fibromuscular dysplasia with balloon angioplasty: a prospective follow-up study. Eur J Vasc Endovasc Surg 2002;23:146-52.

52. Balk E, Raman G, Chung M, et al. Effectiveness of management strategies for renal artery stenosis: a systematic review. Ann Intern Med 2006;145:901-12.

Visceral Artery Disease

Introduction

The visceral arteries, also known as mesenteric arteries and splanchnic arteries, include the celiac artery, superior mesenteric artery (SMA), and inferior mesenteric artery (IMA). These arteries arise from the aorta and supply blood to the gastrointestinal tract, spleen, and liver. The anatomy of the visceral arteries is shown in *Figure 1*.

There are extensive collateral communications between and among the mesenteric arteries. The principal collateral artery between the SMA and IMA is known as the marginal (wandering/meandering) artery of Drummond (*Figure 2*). Chronic mesenteric ischemia (CMI) usually will arise only if at least two of the three arteries are stenotic or occluded.

Epidemiology and Natural History

Large-scale epidemiological studies of mesenteric ischemia are lacking. The incidence of both acute and chronic mesenteric ischemia is likely low. The incidence of CMI is estimated to be 1 per 100,000 cases per year. In an analysis of National Inpatient Sample (NIS) data from 1993 to 1997, only 336 cases of CMI were identified. However, mesenteric artery disease is frequently identified during imaging assessment of patients with atherosclerosis in other vascular beds. The prevalence of mesenteric artery disease may be as high as 70% in patients with coronary artery disease.[1] In a series of 713 patients undergoing angiography for various reasons, mesenteric artery stenosis was found in 17%.[2] The incidence of mesenteric artery stenosis rises with age and approximates 20% in people over the age of 80 years.[3]

The 5-year cardiovascular mortality in patients with CMI has been reported to range from 40-86%.[1] Progression of asymptomatic lesions to symptomatic disease has not been well studied. In a report of 70 patients followed for up to 6 years, four developed symptoms. In a population-based sample from the CHS (Cardiovascular Health Study), 553 patients (average age 77 ± 5 years) underwent mesenteric artery duplex ultrasonography (DUS); of these, 17.5% were found to have stenosis in one or more vessels. At a mean follow-up of 6.5 years, no association between mesenteric artery disease and later development of symptoms, all-cause death, or cardiovascular mortality was found.[4]

Etiology

CMI is most commonly the result of atherosclerosis.[5] Other less common causes include arteriopathies that may result in localized dissection and secondary flow restriction (e.g., fibromuscular dysplasia, segmental arterial mediolysis,[6] Ehlers-Danlos type IV, etc.), vasculitis, radiation, and trauma. These entities should be differentiated from nonocclusive mesenteric ischemia. In this condition, intestinal ischemia is a result of reduced flow to the intestines, often in the setting of acute illness and hypotension.[7] Nonocclusive mesenteric ischemia is usually not associated with reduced blood flow in other major arteries.

Median arcuate ligament syndrome is a disputed cause for CMI-like symptoms. Symptoms in patients with median arcuate ligament

Ido Weinberg, MD, MSc
Consultant Fees/Honoraria:
VIVA Physicians.

Michael R. Jaff, DO, FACC
Consultant Fees/Honoraria: AOPA, Cardinal Health, Covidien, Micell Technologies, Vascular Therapies; Officer, Director, Trustee, or other Fiduciary Role: VIVA Physicians; Other–Non-compensated advisor: Abbott Vascular, Boston Scientific, Cordis, IC Sciences, Medtronic Vascular; Other–Chair, Data Safety and Monitoring Board: Novello; Ownership Interest/Partnership/ Principal: Jana Care, MC10, Northwind Pharmaceuticals, PQ Bypass, Primacea, Sano V, Valiant Medical.

Learner Objectives

Upon completion of this module, the reader will be able to:

1. Recognize that mesenteric ischemia may be the etiology of postprandial abdominal pain and weight loss in patients with systemic atherosclerosis.
2. Select the appropriate imaging study to evaluate patients with suspected mesenteric artery disease.
3. Appreciate that mesenteric vein thrombosis (MVT) accounts for approximately 10% of cases of mesenteric ischemia.
4. Recognize the indications for revascularization for mesenteric ischemia in both the acute and chronic setting.

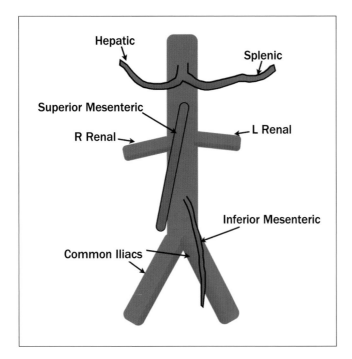

Figure 1
Schematic Depiction of Normal Visceral Artery Anatomy

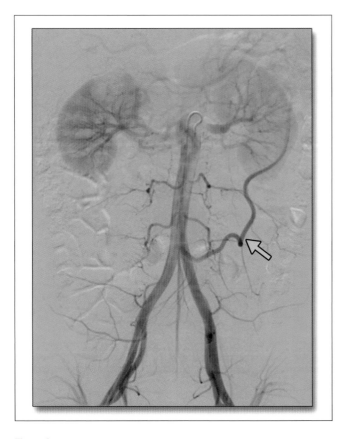

Figure 2
Digital Subtraction Angiogram

The meandering artery of Drummond is marked by the yellow arrow.

syndrome are often hard to differentiate from atherosclerotic CMI, and are postulated to result from celiac artery or celiac plexus compression by the diaphragm.[8] This condition is most commonly encountered in young women.[9]

Acute mesenteric ischemia (AMI) is usually the result of abrupt occlusion due to athero- or thrombo-embolization (e.g., from atrial fibrillation). Most emboli lodge distally in the SMA due to its oblique angle takeoff from the aorta. AMI may also result from acute occlusion of a chronically diseased artery (i.e., complicated aortic atheromatous disease). This process is typically associated with widespread atherosclerosis and affects the artery origin. AMI and malperfusion from branch vessel compromise may complicate the course of aortic dissection.

MVT is an uncommon cause of mesenteric ischemia and accounts for <10% of cases.[10] This condition can be a result of local inflammation (e.g., abdominal surgery, infection, or pancreatitis) or a systemic hypercoagulable condition.[11] It can be easily overlooked if not considered in the differential diagnosis of abdominal pain, and it is recognized on abdominal contrast imaging studies.

Key Point

- Atherosclerosis is the most common cause of visceral artery disease.

Clinical Presentation

CMI classically presents with an insidious onset of postprandial epigastric pain or discomfort, coupled with a sensation of fullness, food avoidance ("fear of food"), and weight loss. While the diagnosis may be straightforward, in hindsight, it is often neglected and delayed given the relatively nonspecific nature of symptoms.[1] The differential diagnosis of abdominal pain is quite broad and includes conditions such as gastritis, peptic ulcer disease, cholecystitis, irritable bowel syndrome, and inflammatory bowel disease.

In contrast, AMI is a medical/surgical emergency, as it may rapidly deteriorate to intestinal gangrene. Embolic occlusion of a mesenteric artery is usually associated with a lack of collaterals; the clinical sequelae of a thrombotic occlusion atop an atherosclerotic plaque in patients with chronic disease may be attenuated by collaterals. Long-term mortality rates of patients with mesenteric ischemia are as high as 70-90%. In an analysis of 4,665 patients in the NIS who underwent intervention for AMI between 2005 and 2009, short-term mortality rates were as high as 40%.[12]

Patients with AMI present with acute, severe abdominal pain, out of proportion to the physical examination findings, diarrhea, and signs of gastrointestinal blood loss, along with laboratory evidence of inflammation and tissue necrosis (e.g., elevated white blood cell counts,

Test	Strength	Limitation
Duplex ultrasonography	Relatively inexpensive, no radiation or contrast	May be limited by obesity and bowel gas; inaccurate for the diagnosis of mesenteric vein thrombosis
Computed tomographic angiography	Accurate, rapid image acquisition	Ionizing radiation, contrast agent exposure
Magnetic resonance angiography	Accurate	Contrast agent (gadolinium) exposure; limited use in patients with claustrophobia and metallic implants; inability to visualize stented segments; requires local experts to produce optimal images
Invasive angiography	Can be combined with a therapeutic procedure, highly accurate	Invasive; exposure to contrast and radiation; risk of embolization or dissection

Table 1
Imaging Tests for Mesenteric Ischemia

erythrocyte sedimentation rates, and C-reactive protein and serum lactate levels).[13]

Patients with MVT have a variable clinical presentation. Asymptomatic MVT is frequently detected on contrast abdominal imaging performed for another indication. Patients with MVT may present either with subacute or acute symptoms of abdominal pain, nausea, and gastrointestinal bleeding. MVT may progress and result in signs of chronic portal hypertension in rare patients.[11]

Key Point

- Symptoms of CMI are often insidious. Classic symptoms include postprandial abdominal pain, food avoidance ("fear of food"), and weight loss.

Diagnosis

Imaging
Multiple imaging modalities can be used to diagnose and follow mesenteric vascular disease. A comparison of imaging tests for mesenteric ischemia is shown in *Table 1*, and a flow diagram suggesting an approach to the diagnosis of visceral artery stenosis is presented in *Figure 3*.

Duplex Ultrasound
The utility of DUS for the diagnosis and surveillance of mesenteric artery disease has been validated in several studies. An SMA peak systolic velocity (PSV) of >300 cm/sec and an end-diastolic velocity (EDV) of >45 cm/sec, respectively, are sensitive and specific for severe stenosis.

Criteria for mesenteric artery in-stent restenosis have been less well validated, and appear to vary from one center to another and from one series to another.[14] The Massachusetts General Hospital criteria for native mesenteric artery stenoses, for example, have been adapted from the Moneta criteria[15] and are presented in *Table 2*. The study is performed after an overnight fast. Also, when celiac artery compression is suspected, measurements of PSV can be repeated during inspiration and expiration (*Figure 4*).

DUS should *not* be a first-line examination in patients with suspected AMI. Also, DUS is not useful in the diagnosis and surveillance of MVT.

Key Point

- DUS, CTA, and MRA are useful for the diagnosis and surveillance of chronic mesenteric artery disease. Duplex scanning is not recommended when AMI is suspected.

Computed Tomographic Angiography and Magnetic Resonance Angiography

Computed tomographic angiography (CTA) provides fast and accurate images of the mesenteric vasculature and can reliably detect findings suggestive of mesenteric ischemia (*Figure 5*). Magnetic resonance angiography (MRA), while accurate for lesions in the ostium of larger vessels, is limited in the assessment of smaller caliber arteries, including much of the IMA. Gadolinium is usually needed

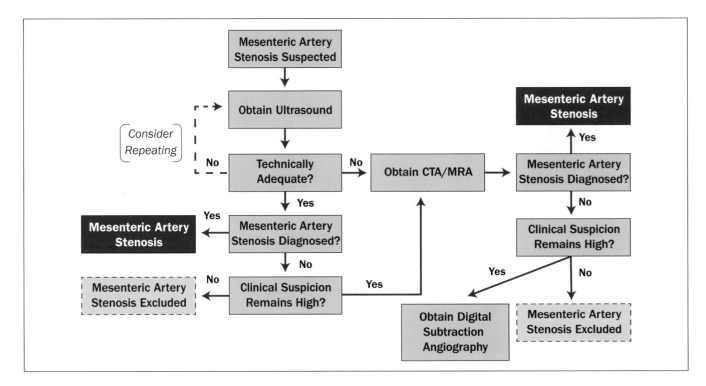

Figure 3
Flow Diagram Suggesting Utilization of Imaging in the Diagnosis of Visceral Artery Stenosis

Artery	>70% Stenosis	Occlusion
Celiac	PSV >250 cm/sec	Absent celiac artery Doppler signal with reversed common hepatic or splenic artery flow
Superior mesenteric	PSV >275 cm/sec	Absent superior mesenteric artery Doppler signal
Inferior mesenteric	PSV >275 cm/sec	Absent inferior mesenteric artery Doppler signal

Table 2
Adapted Moneta Criteria for Native Mesenteric Artery Duplex

PSV = peak systolic velocity.

to provide high-quality images. In the acute setting (e.g., AMI), the lengthy acquisition time associated with MRA limits its usefulness.[16] Also, MRA is not appropriate for evaluation of stented arteries.

CTA and MRA have made it possible to diagnose splanchnic artery pathology that may have gone undetected in the past. Differentiation between clinically significant disease and an incidental finding is not always straightforward. Intervention on the basis of anatomic findings alone is not recommended.[3] There is no ideal objective method for linking symptoms to anatomic findings.

Digital Subtraction Angiography
Before the advent of CTA, digital subtraction angiography (DSA) was considered to be the "gold standard" for evaluation of mesenteric artery anatomy. An advantage of invasive catheterization is the ability to measure a pressure gradient across a visualized stenosis when the anatomic

findings are ambiguous. Cather-based intervention can often proceed during the same sitting. DSA is associated with exposure to contrast, ionizing radiation, and the risk of arterial injury. It also does not visualize extra-arterial anatomy, a possible disadvantage when external arterial compression is suspected.

The American College of Radiology appropriate use criteria recommend CTA as the preferred imaging modality for suspected mesenteric artery disease, followed by DSA and MRA. Focused DUS is also considered in these criteria.[17]

Therapy

Chronic Mesenteric Ischemia
Medical Therapy
Aggressive treatment of atherosclerotic cardiovascular disease risk factors with attention to lipids, blood pressure, and glycemic indices, smoking cessation, and lifestyle is

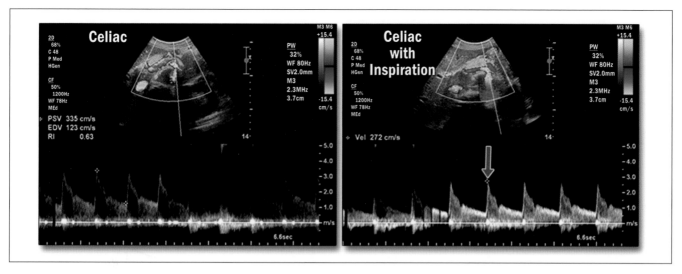

Figure 4

Duplex Ultrasonography Depicting Dynamic Celiac Artery Stenosis

Notice that the peak systolic velocity (PSV, marked by the red arrow) rises with expiration compared with inspiration. This is typical of median arcuate ligament syndrome.

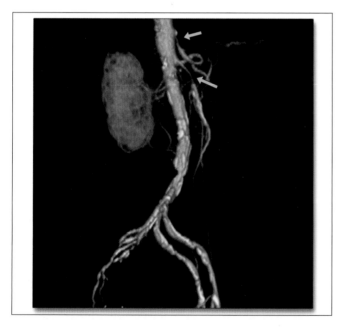

Figure 5

Computed Tomographic Angiography (CTA) Reconstruction of the Abdominal Aorta

CTA reveals significant stenosis in the celiac and in the superior mesenteric arteries (arrows).

the cornerstone of therapy in patients with atherosclerotic visceral artery disease.

No formal dietary recommendations exist for patients with CMI. Nonetheless, as postprandial pain and weight loss are hallmarks of this condition, small frequent meals are often recommended to support adequate caloric intake.

Use of digitalis in patients with atrial fibrillation or heart failure should be discouraged given reports of its association with reduced splanchnic blood flow and nonobstructive mesenteric ischemia. Anticoagulation for patients with atrial fibrillation should be provided in accordance with the CHA_2DS_2-VASc risk score.

Endovascular Therapy

Mesenteric artery atherosclerotic disease usually affects the arterial ostium, and an "endovascular-first" approach is usually offered to symptomatic patients with high-grade disease, if anatomically appropriate. Reports point to favorable short-term outcomes for endovascular therapy in this condition.[18] Stenting is the procedure of choice because aorto-ostial stenoses are difficult to treat with percutaneous transluminal angioplasty alone, due to elastic recoil of the bulky atherosclerotic plaque (*Figure 6*). The technical success rate of endovascular stent revascularization for mesenteric artery stenosis or occlusion exceeds 80%.[19,20] While symptom relief is reported to approach 100% in properly selected cases, restenosis is common and often clinically significant.[21] In a series of 57 patients with CMI who underwent endovascular treatment, 10 required a repeat procedure after an average of 14 months.[19]

There is uncertainty as to the appropriate management of mesenteric artery in-stent restenosis. Some have suggested that covered stents may have the potential for long-term durability.[22,23] Other theoretical approaches for in-stent restenosis may include a drug-eluting stent or a drug-coated balloon. Data regarding long-term patency and the relative efficacy of these approaches are lacking.

Postrevascularization medical management and surveillance methods have not been properly evaluated.

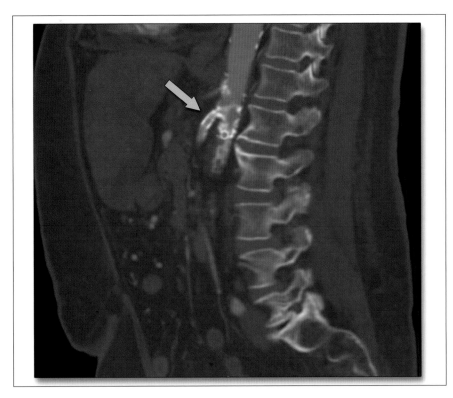

Figure 6

Sagittal Computed Tomographic Angiography (CTA) with Contrast Showing Calcific Atherosclerotic Plaque at Origin of the Superior Mesenteric Artery (SMA)

There is a stent in the SMA (arrow).

Dual antiplatelet therapy for 4 weeks post stenting, followed by long-term antiplatelet monotherapy, is routinely recommended.[1] Reintervention is usually driven by a combination of DUS findings suggestive of restenosis and recurrence of typical CMI-related symptoms. While data are lacking, it is reasonable to follow patients with DUS at 1, 6, and 12 months post procedure and annually thereafter, unless symptoms mandate otherwise.

Surgical Therapy
Surgery for CMI may consist of bypass grafting or trans-aortic endarterectomy. A graft is placed from the aorta to the affected artery, beyond the stenosis. Graft flow is antegrade in the case of a conduit from the thoracic aorta to the mesenteric arteries and retrograde with use of a conduit from the infrarenal aorta or iliac arteries to the mesenteric arteries. The graft can be autologous vein or prosthetic. Symptom relief has been reported in up to 80% of cases.[18] Long-term graft patency rates are largely unavailable. In one report of 98 patients who underwent open surgical bypass for CMI, data were available for 54 patients; stenosis or occlusion occurred in 11 patients over a median of 1.9 years. Older reports suggested high perioperative morbidity and mortality. Endovascular repair has supplanted surgical intervention as the procedure of first choice in patients with appropriate anatomy. Nonetheless, chronic total occlusions are better managed with surgical revascularization.[19]

Acute Mesenteric Ischemia

The goals of treatment in patients with AMI include resuscitation, prevention of disease propagation, prompt resolution of bowel ischemia, and reversal of the inciting event. Resuscitation typically includes delivery of intravenous fluids and broad spectrum antibiotics. Anticoagulation, usually with intravenous unfractionated heparin, should be started in cases of suspected thrombo- or atheroembolization. Mesenteric vasospasm should be targeted either with systemic glucagon or intra-arterial infusion of papaverine or other vasodilators.

Revascularization should be performed promptly. Delayed treatment may result in intestinal ischemia/infarction and sepsis; reperfusion injury may also be worsened if revascularization is delayed.[13] Endovascular revascularization is preferred over surgery, though may not be possible because of time and anatomic constraints.[12,24,25]

Laparotomy and abdominal exploration for bowel ischemia/infarction are integral features of the management of patients with AMI. Diagnosis of AMI is often first made at the time of emergency surgery. Bowel examination/resection and attention to revascularization are the major elements of operation. The latter can include embolectomy and/or bypass. Second-look surgery is usually recommended, as the initial intraoperative assessment of the extent of bowel ischemia can be inaccurate.

Mesenteric Vein Thrombosis

Treatment of MVT with anticoagulation is aimed at preventing mesenteric ischemia in the short term and preventing thrombosis recurrence in the long term. Ischemia-related gastrointestinal bleeding should not prevent treatment with an anticoagulant when possible. Adjunctive therapies sometimes may be needed. For patients with at-risk bowel, endovascular infusion of a vasodilator or thrombolytic agent may enhance bowel perfusion,[26] though this practice is controversial.[13] For patients in whom there are already signs of peritonitis, surgical exploration is necessary.

Key Points

- Aggressive treatment of atherosclerotic cardiovascular disease risk factors with attention to lipids, blood pressure, glycemic indices, smoking cessation, and lifestyle is the cornerstone of therapy in patients with atherosclerotic visceral artery disease.

- Patients with visceral artery disease should be treated with guideline-directed medical therapy for secondary prevention, and their risk factors should be optimized.

- For patients with symptoms of CMI and weight loss, revascularization is required when anatomically feasible.

- Given the morbidity and mortality of surgical therapy, endovascular therapy with stenting is used increasingly as the initial approach in patients with CMI.

- For patients presenting with AMI, revascularization should be performed promptly to avoid bowel infarction and sepsis. In these cases, endovascular revascularization prior to intestinal surgery is preferred, though may not be possible because of time and anatomic constraints.

References

1. Zeller T, Rastan A, Sixt S. Chronic atherosclerotic mesenteric ischemia (CMI). Vasc Med 2010;15:333-8.

2. Bron KM, Redman HC. Splanchnic artery stenosis and occlusion. Incidence; arteriographic and clinical manifestations. Radiology 1969;92:323-8.

3. Mensink PB, van Petersen AS, Geelkerken RH, Otte JA, Huisman AB, Kolkman JJ. Clinical significance of splanchnic artery stenosis. Br J Surg 2006;93:1377-82.

4. Wilson DB, Mostafavi K, Craven TE, Ayerdi J, Edwards MS, Hansen KJ. Clinical course of mesenteric artery stenosis in elderly Americans. Arch Intern Med 2006;166:2095-100.

5. Paterno F, Longo WE. The etiology and pathogenesis of vascular disorders of the intestine. Radiol Clin North Am 2008;46:877-85.

6. Kalva SP, Somarouthu B, Jaff MR, Wicky S. Segmental arterial mediolysis: clinical and imaging features at presentation and during follow-up. J Vasc Interv Radiol 2011; 22:1380-7.

7. Reginelli A, Iacobellis F, Berritto D, et al. Mesenteric ischemia: the importance of differential diagnosis for the surgeon. BMC Surg 2013;13:S51.

8. Jimenez JC, Harlander-Locke M, Dutson EP. Open and laparoscopic treatment of median arcuate ligament syndrome. J Vasc Surg 2012;56:869-73.

9. Sadiq IR, Abdulbaki A, Azemi T. Median arcuate ligament syndrome: use of fractional flow reserve in documentation of chronic mesenteric ischemia. Vasc Med 2014;19:317-21.

10. Harnik IG, Brandt LJ. Mesenteric venous thrombosis. Vasc Med 2010;15:407-18.

11. Singal AK, Kamath PS, Tefferi A. Mesenteric venous thrombosis. Mayo Clinic Proc 2013;88:285-94.

12. Beaulieu RJ, Arnaoutakis KD, Abularrage CJ, Efron DT, Schneider E, Black JH 3rd. Comparison of open and endovascular treatment of acute mesenteric ischemia. J Vasc Surg 2014;59:159-64

13. Oldenburg WA, Lau LL, Rodenberg TJ, Edmonds HJ, Burger CD. Acute mesenteric ischemia: a clinical review. Arch Intern Med 2004;164:1054-62.

14. AbuRahma AF, Stone PA, Srivastava M, et al. Mesenteric/celiac duplex ultrasound interpretation criteria revisited. J Vasc Surg 2012;55:428-62.

15. Moneta GL, Yeager RA, Dalman R, Antonovic R, Hall LD, Porter JM. Duplex ultrasound criteria for diagnosis of splanchnic artery stenosis or occlusion. J Vasc Surg 1991;14:511-8.

16. Costa AF, Chidambaram V, Lee JJ, Asquith J, Skaff ER, Thipphavong S. Multidetector computed tomography of mesenteric ischaemia. Insights Imaging 2014;5:657-66.

17. Oliva IB, Davarpanah AH, Rybicki FJ, et al. ACR Appropriateness Criteria ® imaging of mesenteric ischemia. Abdom Imaging 2013;38:714-9.

18. Schermerhorn ML, Giles KA, Hamdan AD, Wyers MC, Pomposelli FB. Mesenteric revascularization: management and outcomes in the United States, 1988-2006. J Vasc Surg 2009;50:341-8.

19. Silva JA, White CJ, Collins TJ, et al. Endovascular therapy for chronic mesenteric ischemia. J Am Coll Cardiol 2006;47:944-50.

20. Zeller T, Rastan A, Schwarzwalder U, et al. Endovascular therapy of chronic mesenteric ischaemia. Eurointervention 2007;2:444-51.

21. Schaefer PJ, Schaefer FK, Mueller-Huelsbeck S, Jahnke T. Chronic mesenteric ischemia: stenting of mesenteric arteries. Abdom Imaging 2007;32:304-9.

22. Margiotta A, Gray BH. Assessment of recurrent mesenteric ischemia after stenting with a pressure wire. Vasc Med 2014;19:137-41.

23. Oderich GS, Erdoes LS, Lesar C, et al. Comparison of covered stents versus bare metal stents for treatment of chronic atherosclerotic mesenteric arterial disease. J Vasc Surg 2013;58:1316-23.

24. Acosta S, Björck M. Modern treatment of acute mesenteric ischaemia. Br J Surg 2014;101:e100-8.

25. Block TA, Acosta S, Björck M. Endovascular and open surgery for acute occlusion of the superior mesenteric artery. J Vasc Surg 2010;52;959-66.

26. Hollingshead M, Burke CT, Mauro MA, Weeks SM, Dixon RG, Jaques PF. Transcatheter thrombolytic therapy for acute mesenteric and portal vein thrombosis. J Vasc Interv Radiol 2005;16:651-61.

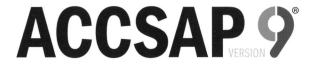

Adult Clinical Cardiology Self-Assessment Program

Book 6

Vascular Diseases

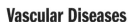

CAROTID ARTERY DISEASE, STROKE/TIA

Editor:

Patrick T. O'Gara, MD, MACC

This author has nothing to disclose.

Stroke Overview

Todd S. Perlstein, MD

Mohammed Teleb, MD

Please refer to the online version of ACCSAP 9 to learn about this topic.

Extracranial Carotid Artery Disease

Todd S. Perlstein, MD

Please refer to the online version of ACCSAP 9 to learn about this topic.

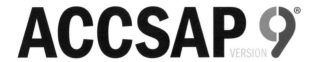

ACCSAP 9 VERSION®

Adult Clinical Cardiology Self-Assessment Program

Book 6
Vascular Diseases

VENOUS THROMBOEMBOLIC DISEASE

Editor:

Patrick T. O'Gara, MD, MACC
This author has nothing to disclose.

Venous Thromboembolic Disease   **157**
Gregory Piazza, MD, FACC

Venous Thromboembolic Disease

Introduction

Venous thromboembolism (VTE), including deep vein thrombosis (DVT) and PE, is the third most common cardiovascular cause of morbidity and mortality after myocardial infarction (MI) and stroke. DVT and PE may result in debilitating long-term complications of post-thrombotic syndrome[1] and chronic thromboembolic pulmonary hypertension,[2] respectively. Patients with VTE and its sequelae constitute an increasing proportion of inpatient consultations and outpatient referrals in cardiovascular medicine practice.

> ### Key Point
>
> - VTE, including DVT and PE, is the third most common cause of cardiovascular morbidity and mortality after MI and stroke.

Epidemiology

In a population-based analysis of 5,025 central Massachusetts residents, age- and sex-adjusted annual event rates for initial VTE increased from 73/100,000 in 1985-1986 to 133/100,000 in 2009, primarily due to an increase in PE.[3]

In another epidemiological study of data from 1998 and 2005, the number of patients with primary or secondary PE on hospital discharge increased from 126,546 to 229,637, while the hospital case fatality rate decreased from 12.3% to 8.2%.[4] An analysis of the Danish National Registry of Patients demonstrated that patients with an initial episode of VTE have an increased mortality over 30 years of follow-up.[5] Recurrent PE was an important cause of increased mortality.

Risk Factors

Risk factors for VTE include lifestyle-related conditions, inherited thrombophilias, acquired disorders of endothelial injury, stasis, hypercoagulability, and inflammation (*Table 1*). The majority of VTE patients present with a combination of risk factors.

Lifestyle
Smoking is a potent VTE risk factor, especially in women. Obesity doubles the risk of VTE. Diets that limit red meat consumption and are rich in fish and vegetables lower the risk of VTE. Persistently high stress levels increase the risk of PE.

Inherited
Major inherited thrombophilias include factor V Leiden, prothrombin gene mutation 20210, and deficiencies of protein C, protein S, or antithrombin. Prevalence of inherited thrombophilias varies by population. Testing for hypercoagulable states should be reserved for patients in whom there is a high suspicion and in whom the results of the evaluation will impact therapy.[6] Inherited thrombophilias are frequently suspected in patients with VTE at a young age, multiple family members with VTE, idiopathic or recurrent VTE, or recurrent pregnancy losses.

Gregory Piazza, MD, FACC
Research/Research Grants: BMS, Daiichi Sankyo, EKOS, Janssen Pharmaceuticals, Thrombosis Research Institute.

Learner Objectives

Upon completion of this module, the reader will be able to:

1. Recognize risk factors for venous thromboembolism (VTE) so that vulnerable patients are identified.
2. Use diagnostic algorithms for patients with suspected VTE to avoid delays in recognizing the disease.
3. Employ a risk stratification algorithm for patients with acute pulmonary embolism (PE) to identify those who may benefit from advanced therapies.
4. Select therapeutic options for patients with VTE so that adverse outcomes, recurrent episodes, and disease sequelae are avoided.
5. Recommend appropriate prophylactic strategies for at-risk patients to prevent VTE.

Acquired

Acquired risk factors are far more common than inherited thrombophilias. Advanced age, malignancy, immobility, and recent trauma, surgery, or hospitalization are well-recognized risk factors. The lupus anticoagulant, antiphospholipid antibodies, and anticardiolipin antibodies are potent acquired risk factors for VTE. VTE is an important women's health concern. Pregnancy, hormonal contraceptive techniques, and hormone replacement therapy are important VTE risk factors. Chronic medical conditions, such as heart failure and chronic obstructive pulmonary disease, also contribute to the risk of VTE. Atherosclerosis and VTE share common pathophysiological processes of inflammation, hypercoagulability, and endothelial injury.[7] Accordingly, atherosclerotic cardiovascular disease and its risk factors are now recognized as important risk factors for VTE.

Inflammatory

The role of inflammation as a risk factor for VTE has long been suspected, based on the observation of an increased frequency of DVT and PE in patients with chronic inflammatory disorders such as rheumatoid arthritis and inflammatory bowel disease.[7] Elevations in C-reactive protein (CRP), a sensitive marker of systemic inflammation, have been linked to an increased risk of VTE.[8] In the JUPITER (Justification for the Use of Statins in Prevention: an Intervention Trial Evaluating Rosuvastatin) trial, healthy men and women with both low-density lipoprotein cholesterol levels of <130 mg/dl and high-sensitivity CRP levels of ≥2.0 mg/L had significant reductions in symptomatic VTE when randomized to therapy with rosuvastatin.[9]

Lifestyle
- Smoking
- Obesity
- Diet (high red meat, low fish and vegetable consumption)
- Stress

Inherited
- Factor V Leiden
- Prothrombin gene mutation 20210
- Deficiencies of protein C, protein S, or antithrombin
- Family history of venous thromboembolism (VTE)

Acquired
- Advancing age
- Malignancy
- Pregnancy, hormonal contraception, or hormone replacement therapy
- Atherosclerotic cardiovascular disease and risk-associated factors (including diabetes, dyslipidemia, hypertension)
- Chronic medical illness (including heart failure, chronic obstructive pulmonary disease, chronic kidney disease)
- Immobility
- Recent history of trauma, surgery, or hospitalization
- Personal history of VTE
- Lupus anticoagulant, antiphospholipid antibodies, or anticardiolipin antibodies
- Hyperhomocysteinemia (less commonly inherited secondary to a mutation in methylenetetrahydrofolate reductase)
- Long-haul air travel
- Pacemaker or implantable cardiac defibrillator leads and indwelling venous catheters

Inflammatory
- Acute infectious illness
- Blood transfusion and erythropoiesis-stimulating agents
- Chronic inflammation (including systemic vasculitides, inflammatory bowel disease)

Table 1

Risk Factors for Venous Thromboembolism

Key Point

- VTE shares common pathophysiology and risk factors (such as inflammation, hypertension, dyslipidemia, obesity, and smoking) with atherothrombosis.

Pathophysiology

Deep Vein Thrombosis

DVT results from a combination of pathophysiological states, including endothelial injury, stasis, inflammation, and hypercoagulability. Although the deep veins of the lower extremity are the most common site for formation of DVT, thrombosis may also develop within the deep veins of the upper extremities, abdomen, and pelvis. The May-Thurner syndrome (extrinsic compression of the left common iliac vein by the right common iliac artery) should be considered in a young adult with left leg swelling and DVT.

Pulmonary Embolism

Thrombi usually originate from the deep venous system of the lower extremities and pelvis, embolize through the inferior vena cava (IVC) and right heart, and obstruct the pulmonary arterial tree, thereby causing hemodynamic and gas exchange abnormalities. Direct physical obstruction of the pulmonary arteries, hypoxemia, and release of potent pulmonary arterial vasoconstrictors increase pulmonary vascular resistance and right ventricular (RV) afterload.[10] Acute RV pressure overload may result in RV hypokinesis and dilation, tricuspid regurgitation, and ultimately, right heart failure. Patients with acute PE and RV failure may decompensate and develop systemic arterial hypotension, cardiogenic shock, and cardiac arrest. Increased RV diastolic pressure causes deviation of the interventricular septum toward

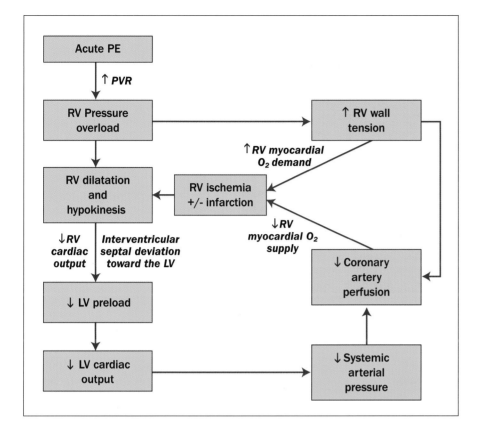

Figure 1
Pathways to RV Pathology

The pathophysiology of RV dysfunction due to acute PE.

LV = left ventricular; PE = pulmonary embolism; PVR = pulmonary vascular resistance; RV = right ventricular.

the left ventricle (LV) and impairs LV preload. RV pressure overload may also result in increased wall stress and ischemia by increasing myocardial oxygen demand while simultaneously limiting its supply (*Figure 1*). Mismatch between myocardial oxygen demand and supply may result in RV ischemia and infarction.

Gas exchange abnormalities in patients with acute PE most often result from a combination of ventilation-to-perfusion mismatch, increases in total dead space, and right-to-left shunting.

Key Points

- The May-Thurner syndrome should be recognized clinically in a young adult with left leg swelling and DVT from extrinsic compression of the left common iliac vein by the right common iliac artery.

- In a subset of patients, PE causes acute RV pressure overload, which may culminate in RV failure, systemic arterial hypotension, cardiogenic shock, and death.

Diagnosis of Deep Vein Thrombosis

Clinical Presentation
Although most often observed in the lower extremities, DVT may also develop in the upper extremities, especially in the setting of chronically indwelling central venous foreign bodies, such as catheters, and in syndromes of thoracic outlet obstruction. Patients with lower extremity DVT will typically report a cramping or pulling sensation of the calf or thigh that worsens with ambulation. Patients may also note swelling or asymmetry in the size of their legs. Physical examination findings include warmth, edema, and tenderness of the extremity.

Laboratory Testing
Plasma D-dimer is a nonspecific marker of endogenous fibrinolysis. It is elevated in VTE, as well as many other systemic illnesses and conditions, such as MI, heart failure, infection, surgery, aortic dissection, and pregnancy. D-dimer has the greatest utility in evaluation of outpatients or emergency department patients with suspected VTE because many inpatients will have elevated levels due to other conditions.

D-dimer offers the greatest accuracy for suspected DVT when used in combination with an assessment of pretest clinical likelihood. In patients with low pretest clinical probability, a negative D-dimer can exclude the diagnosis of DVT without further testing, such as venous ultrasound. Among patients with higher clinical suspicion for DVT, further evaluation is often warranted despite negative D-dimer results.

Imaging
Venous ultrasound is the initial imaging test of choice for evaluation of suspected lower or upper extremity DVT. Failure to compress a vein is diagnostic of DVT (*Figure 2*). Anatomical constraints limit ultrasonographic evaluation of the pelvic veins and upper extremity veins proximal to the clavicle.

Alternative imaging modalities for evaluation of suspected DVT include computed tomography (CT), magnetic resonance (MR), and invasive contrast venography. These techniques are generally reserved for imaging venous segments that are inadequately assessed by venous ultrasound.

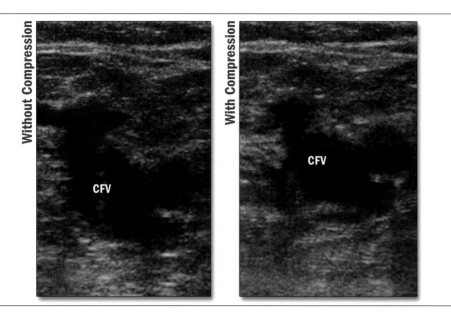

Figure 2
Venous Ultrasonography Demonstrating Noncompressibility of the Left CFV, Consistent With DVT

CFV = common femoral vein; DVT = deep vein thrombosis.

Overall Diagnostic Algorithm

An algorithm for evaluation of suspected DVT combines an assessment of pretest clinical probability, D-dimer testing, and imaging when appropriate (*Figure 3*).

Diagnosis of Pulmonary Embolism

Clinical Presentation

Dyspnea is the most frequently reported symptom. On physical examination, tachypnea is the most common sign. PE patients may also exhibit signs of RV failure such as tachycardia, distended neck veins, tricuspid regurgitation, and accentuation of the pulmonic valve closure sound (P_2).

Laboratory Testing

D-dimer testing is most helpful in patients with suspected PE who present as outpatients or in the emergency department. Because of its high negative predictive value, the D-dimer enzyme-linked immunosorbent assay (ELISA) can be used to exclude PE in outpatients with low to moderate pretest probability without the need for further costly testing. Inpatients should proceed directly to imaging as the initial test for PE because many will already have elevated D-dimers due to comorbid illness.

Electrocardiogram

The electrocardiogram (ECG) may suggest alternative diagnoses such as MI. The ECG may also demonstrate findings suggestive of RV strain due to PE (*Table 2*). Some patients may simply demonstrate signs of increased adrenergic tone with resting sinus tachycardia.

Imaging

Like the ECG, the chest X-ray may suggest alternative diagnoses such as pneumonia. A normal or near-normal chest X-ray in a patient with dyspnea or hypoxemia suggests PE. The majority of patients with PE will have some abnormality, such as cardiomegaly or pleural effusion, on the chest X-ray.

Contrast-enhanced chest CT has emerged as the dominant diagnostic imaging technique to evaluate suspected PE (*Figure 4*). In general, ventilation-perfusion (V/Q) lung scans are reserved for patients with major renal impairment, anaphylaxis to intravenous iodinated contrast, or pregnancy. Although a high probability scan in the setting of moderate to high pretest clinical suspicion virtually guarantees the diagnosis, and a normal scan excludes it, the majority of patients have intermediate or indeterminate probability scans requiring further imaging.

MR angiography has shown limited sensitivity in the diagnosis of acute PE. Invasive contrast pulmonary angiography is reserved for the rare circumstance in which other imaging modalities are nondiagnostic, and a high pretest clinical suspicion persists. Although insensitive for diagnosis, transthoracic echocardiography is superb for detecting RV dysfunction in the setting of pressure overload and serves an important role in risk stratification of patients with proven acute PE. Transesophageal echocardiography may be useful for diagnosis of proximal PE, especially in critically ill patients who cannot safely be transported.

Overall Diagnostic Algorithm

Diagnostic algorithms that integrate an assessment of pretest clinical probability with appropriate use of D-dimer testing and imaging allow management decisions to be made efficiently and safely in the vast majority of patients with suspected PE (*Figure 5*).

> **Key Point**
>
> - Algorithms for diagnosis of DVT and PE offer the greatest accuracy when incorporating an assessment of pretest clinical probability with appropriate use of D-dimer testing and imaging.

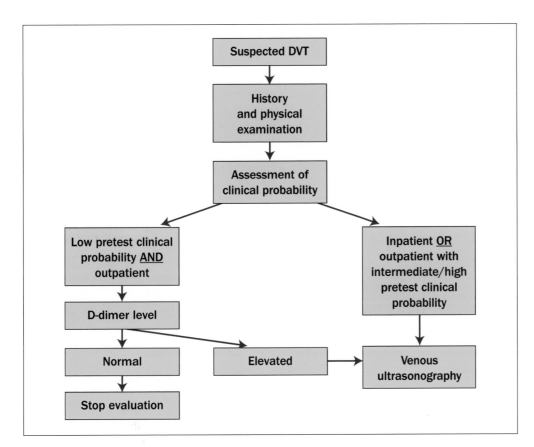

Figure 3

Overall Diagnostic Algorithm for Evaluation of Possible Deep Vein Thrombosis (DVT)

Risk Stratification for Pulmonary Embolism

While the clinical presentation of hemodynamic instability defines massive PE, detection of RV dysfunction identifies normotensive patients with submassive PE. RV dysfunction in patients with PE has been associated with increased 30-day mortality and risk of VTE recurrence.[10] Clinical examination, ECG, cardiac biomarkers, chest CT, and echocardiography are important tools for detection of RV dysfunction (*Figure 6*). Risk stratification to detect RV dysfunction in patients with PE is critical to identify those who might benefit from advanced therapies such as fibrinolysis, catheter-assisted "pharmacomechanical" embolectomy, or surgery.

Physical examination findings of RV failure and ECG evidence of RV strain are rapid and inexpensive indicators of submassive PE. Elevations in cardiac biomarkers, including troponin and B-type natriuretic peptide (BNP) are associated with RV dysfunction and identify patients with submassive PE.[10] Detection of RV enlargement on chest CT, defined as an RV diameter to LV diameter ratio of >0.9, predicts increased PE-related mortality.[11] Chest CT is especially useful because these ratios are acquired during the initial diagnostic scan and require no additional imaging.

Echocardiography remains the imaging technique of choice for detection of RV dysfunction in the setting of PE and identification of submassive PE patients. Characteristic echocardiographic findings in patients with submassive PE include RV dilatation and hypokinesis, interventricular

- Sinus tachycardia

- Incomplete or complete right bundle branch block

- T-wave inversions in leads V_1-V_4

- S wave in lead I and a Q-wave and T-wave inversion in lead III (S1Q3T3)

- Atrial fibrillation

Table 2

Major Electrocardiographic Findings of Acute Pulmonary Embolism

septal flattening and paradoxical motion toward the LV, abnormal transmitral Doppler flow profile (represented by the A wave making a greater contribution to LV diastolic filling than the E wave), tricuspid regurgitation, pulmonary hypertension (identified by a peak tricuspid regurgitant jet velocity >2.6 m/sec) and loss of inspiratory collapse of the IVC (*Table 3*). The finding of severe RV free wall hypokinesis and apical sparing (McConnell sign) is specific for acute PE. Echocardiography should be performed in patients with acute PE and clinical evidence of RV failure, elevated levels of cardiac biomarkers, or unexpected clinical decompensation.

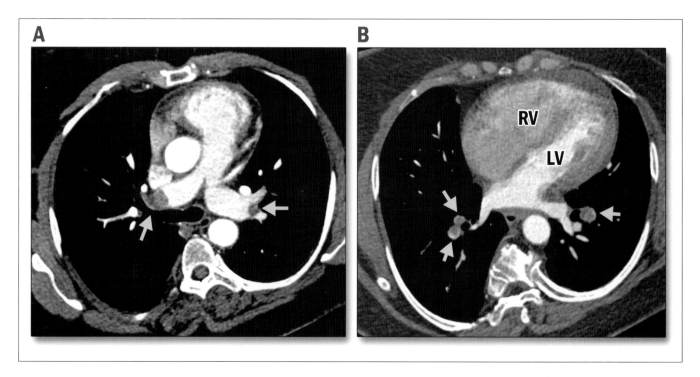

Figure 4

CT Scan Finds Filling Defects, PEs

Contrast-enhanced chest CT demonstrating filling defects (arrows) in both main pulmonary arteries consistent with bilateral PE (**panel A**). The diameter of the RV exceeds that of the LV, consistent with RV enlargement and submassive PE (**panel B**). Multiple segmental PEs (arrows) are also noted distally (**panel B**).

CT = computed tomography; LV = left ventricle; PE = pulmonary embolism; RV = right ventricle.

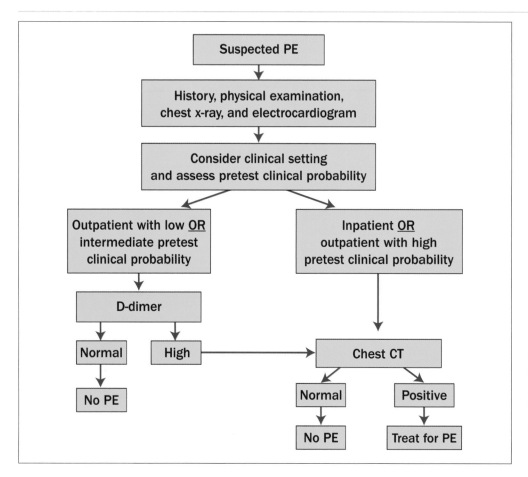

Figure 5

An Integrated Diagnostic Algorithm for Patients With Suspected PE

CT = computed tomography; PE = pulmonary embolism.

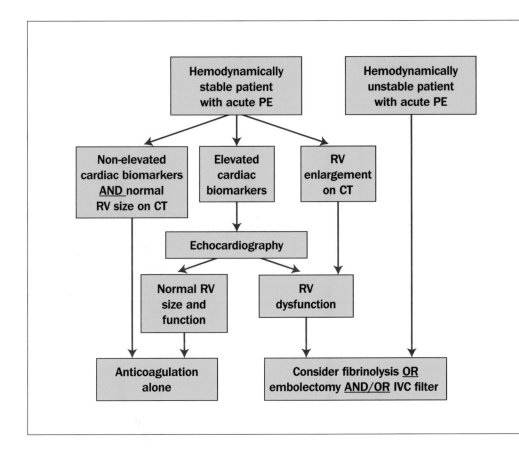

Figure 6

An Algorithm for Risk Stratification of Patients With Acute PE

CT = computed tomography; IVC = inferior vena cava; PE = pulmonary embolism; RV = right ventricular.

- Right ventricular (RV) dilation and hypokinesis

- Systolic interventricular septal flattening and paradoxical motion toward the left ventricle (LV)

- Increased RV diastolic diameter-to-LV diastolic diameter ratio

- Tricuspid regurgitation

- Pulmonary hypertension as identified by a tricuspid regurgitant jet velocity >2.6 m/s

- Dilation and loss of collapse of the inferior vena cava with inspiration

- Decrease in tricuspid annular plane systolic excursion (TAPSE) <17 mm

Table 3

Major Echocardiographic Findings of Acute Pulmonary Embolism

Key Point

- Risk stratification to detect RV dysfunction in patients with PE is critical to identify those who might benefit from advanced therapies, such as fibrinolysis, catheter-assisted "pharmacomechanical" embolectomy, or surgery.

Management of Venous Thromboembolism

Spectrum of Disease

DVT encompasses a wide spectrum of disease, including phlegmasia cerulea dolens and iliofemoral, proximal lower extremity, isolated calf, and upper extremity DVT.

Phlegmasia cerulea dolens and iliofemoral DVT may result in increased risk of post-thrombotic syndrome. Pelvic vein thrombosis describes DVT of the IVC; gonadal veins; and common, internal, and external iliac veins. Superior vena cava syndrome may complicate upper extremity DVT in the setting of chronic indwelling venous foreign bodies, such as an infusion catheter, pacemaker, or defibrillator leads.

Acute PE comprises a number of clinical syndromes, including massive PE, submassive PE, and PE with normal blood pressure and preserved RV function. Massive PE describes a subset of PE patients who present with syncope, hypotension, cardiogenic shock, or cardiac arrest. Normotensive patients with acute PE and evidence of RV dysfunction have submassive PE, and an increased risk of adverse events and early mortality.[10]

	Warfarin	NOACs
Onset of action	Slow	Rapid
Dosing	Variable	Fixed
Drug–food effect	Yes	No
Drug–drug interactions	Many	Few
Routine laboratory monitoring	Yes	No
Half-life	Long	Short
Reversal agent available	Yes	Yes*

Table 4

Major Differences Between Warfarin, Non-Vitamin K Oral Anticoagulants (NOACs)

*Idarucizumab is approved by the US FDA for patients treated with dabigatran (Pradaxa) when reversal of the anticoagulant effects of dabigatran is needed for emergency surgery/urgent procedures, or in life-threatening or uncontrolled bleeding. A reversal agent for the direct factor Xa inhibitors, rivaroxaban, apixaban, and edoxaban, has not been US FDA approved.

Anticoagulation

Anticoagulation is the cornerstone of therapy for patients with VTE regardless of whether advanced therapies are also indicated. Currently, US Food and Drug Administration (FDA)-approved agents for VTE include unfractionated heparin (UFH), low molecular weight heparin (LMWH), fondaparinux, argatroban, bivalirudin, warfarin, and the nonvitamin K oral anticoagulants (NOACs) rivaroxaban, dabigatran, apixaban, and edoxaban.

Immediate anticoagulation with intravenous UFH is administered as a bolus followed by continuous infusion and titrated to a goal activated partial thromboplastin time (aPTT) of 2-3 times the upper limit of normal, or approximately 60-80 seconds. Weight-based heparin nomograms help to rapidly achieve therapeutic levels of anticoagulation. Because it can be discontinued and rapidly reversed, intravenous UFH is favored for patients undergoing advanced therapies for VTE, such as fibrinolysis, catheter-based intervention, or surgery.

LMWHs are dosed according to weight and renal function, administered subcutaneously, and do not require routine dose adjustment or laboratory monitoring. LMWHs are at least as safe and effective as UFH for immediate anticoagulation and transition to oral anticoagulation after acute VTE. LMWH monotherapy without transition to oral anticoagulation halves the risk of VTE recurrence compared with warfarin in patients with active cancer.[12] Although UFH is largely eliminated by the liver, LMWHs are cleared renally. Whereas the effects of UFH can be fully reversed with protamine, the effects of LMWHs are only partially reversed with this agent.

Fondaparinux, a synthetic pentasaccharide, has been shown to be as safe and effective as LMWHs in treatment of DVT and intravenous UFH in the treatment of acute PE. Fondaparinux is administered subcutaneously in fixed once-daily doses according to weight, and does not require routine monitoring or dose adjustment. Like LMWHs, fondaparinux is cleared by the kidneys. In contrast to UFH and LMWHs, fondaparinux is not associated with heparin-induced thrombocytopenia (HIT).

Until the introduction of the NOACs, warfarin had been the default therapy for outpatient oral anticoagulation for VTE. Although a growing number of VTE patients are being prescribed NOACs, warfarin continues to be an important option in the anticoagulation armamentarium. Oral anticoagulation with warfarin is overlapped with heparin, LMWH, or fondaparinux for a *minimum of 5 days* until full therapeutic efficacy is achieved. For the majority of patients with VTE, the target international normalized ratio (INR) range is 2-3.

Warfarin management is challenging because of many drug-food, drug-alcohol, and drug-drug interactions, and genetic polymorphisms that impact its metabolism. Dosing algorithms that incorporate pharmacogenetic testing have not improved the safety and efficacy of warfarin anticoagulation in large randomized controlled trials.[13-15] Anticoagulation management services facilitate INR testing, dose adjustment, and clinical monitoring of patients prescribed warfarin.

NOACs offer several advantages over warfarin for oral anticoagulation in VTE patients (*Table 4*). Dabigatran, rivaroxaban, apixaban, and edoxaban have been shown to be safe and effective for oral anticoagulation for VTE, and are all FDA-approved.[16-21] Compared with warfarin, the NOACs have demonstrated both noninferiority for prevention of recurrent venous thromboembolic events and improved safety (*Table 5*).

Agent	Administration*	Efficacy Compared with Warfarin	Safety Compared with Warfarin	Extended-duration Anticoagulation for Prevention of Recurrence After Unprovoked VTE
Dabigatran	Initial therapy with a parenteral agent, then switch to dabigatran	Noninferior for recurrent VTE or VTE-related death	↔ major bleeding	↓ 93% vs. placebo Noninferior vs. warfarin (INR 2-3)
Rivaroxaban	Oral loading dose 15 mg twice daily for 3 weeks, then 20 mg daily	Noninferior for recurrent VTE	↓ major bleeding	↓ 82% vs. placebo
Apixaban	Oral loading dose 10 mg twice daily for 1 week, then 5 mg twice daily; 2.5 mg twice daily is an option for long-term prevention of recurrent VTE	Noninferior for recurrent VTE or VTE-related death	↓ major bleeding	↓ 81% vs. placebo
Edoxaban	Initial therapy with a parenteral agent, then switch to edoxaban	Noninferior for recurrent VTE	↓ major bleeding	—

Table 5

Novel Oral Anticoagulants for Treatment of Acute Venous Thromboembolism (VTE)

*Standard dosing. Dose adjustment may be required for advanced age, low body weight, and impaired renal function.

INR = international normalized ratio.

Dabigatran and edoxaban are administered in fixed doses after at least 5 days of parenteral anticoagulation with UFH, LMWHs, fondaparinux, or a direct thrombin inhibitor. Rivaroxaban and apixaban are administered as completely oral monotherapy with a fixed loading dose followed by a maintenance dose. All of the NOACs rely upon renal clearance to some extent.

Advanced Therapy for Deep Vein Thrombosis

Advanced therapy is considered for patients with proximal upper extremity or iliofemoral DVT, especially in young, otherwise healthy patients with severe symptoms. Fibrinolysis should be catheter-directed to gain access to the obstructed deep venous system. The National Heart, Lung, and Blood Institute (NHLBI)-sponsored ATTRACT (Acute Venous Thrombosis: Thrombus Removal with Adjunctive Catheter-Directed Thrombolysis) trial has completed enrollment and will determine if catheter-based fibrinolytic therapy can safely prevent post-thrombotic syndrome and improve quality of life in patients with proximal DVT. Surgical thrombectomy is considered in patients with massive or severely symptomatic DVT in whom fibrinolysis has failed or is contraindicated.

Advanced Therapy for Pulmonary Embolism

Consensus guidelines[22-24] recommend advanced therapy for patients with massive PE. Advanced therapy such as systemic fibrinolysis is considered for normotensive PE patients with severe RV dysfunction or major myocardial necrosis (submassive PE)[22] or both imaging evidence of RV dysfunction and elevated cardiac troponin (intermediate- to high-risk PE).[24] Options for advanced therapy for treatment of PE include systemic fibrinolysis, catheter-assisted "pharmacomechanical" therapy, and surgical pulmonary embolectomy.

The FDA has approved recombinant tissue plasminogen activator (t-PA) 100 mg administered as a continuous infusion over 2 hours for fibrinolysis of acute PE. The goals of fibrinolysis are rapid reduction in RV pressure overload, stabilization of hemodynamics, and normalization of gas exchange. All patients being considered for fibrinolysis require meticulous screening for contraindications that make the bleeding risk prohibitive. Intracranial hemorrhage is the most severe and feared complication of fibrinolytic therapy.

In the largest study of full-dose systemic fibrinolysis, tenecteplase reduced the risk of death or cardiovascular collapse by 56% in 1,006 submassive PE patients.[25] However, this benefit was offset by a nearly fivefold increased risk of major bleeding and a tenfold increased risk of hemorrhagic stroke. Meta-analyses of trials of systemic fibrinolysis for acute PE have demonstrated similar findings.[26,27]

Concern over the risk of major bleeding, especially intracranial hemorrhage, has sparked interest in alternative advanced therapies with lower bleeding risk, such as catheter-assisted embolectomy or surgical embolectomy. Catheter-assisted embolectomy is an emerging technique that combines low-dose "local" fibrinolysis and mechanical thrombus disruption. One such technique, ultrasound-facilitated, catheter-directed, low-dose fibrinolysis, requires only a fraction of the systemic fibrinolytic dose and rapidly improves RV function while minimizing the risk of intracranial hemorrhage.[28,29] Ultrasound-facilitated, catheter-based, low-dose fibrinolysis is FDA-approved for treatment of PE.

Surgical pulmonary embolectomy is indicated for patients in whom fibrinolysis or catheter-based techniques have failed or are contraindicated, as well as for those with paradoxical embolism, persistent right heart thrombi, and "clot-in-transit."[30] Surgical pulmonary embolectomy requires a median sternotomy and cardiopulmonary bypass, and is most successful in patients with large, centrally located thrombi.

Inferior Vena Cava Filters
IVC filter insertion is considered for patients with massive or submassive PE in whom fibrinolysis and surgical pulmonary embolectomy are contraindicated or unavailable. IVC filters are also indicated for patients in whom standard anticoagulation is contraindicated, such as in those with active bleeding. In a randomized trial, IVC filter insertion for patients with acute PE who were anticoagulated did not reduce the risk of symptomatic recurrence compared with anticoagulation alone.[31]

IVC filters reduce the risk of PE in the short term, but appear to increase the risk of DVT in the long term. Retrievable IVC filters provide a safe and effective alternative to permanent filters and should be removed in patients with only transient contraindications to anticoagulation, such as the need for noncardiac surgery with acute DVT. Neurosurgical patients with DVT frequently require this approach.

Pulmonary Embolism Response Teams
Multidisciplinary PE Response Teams merge the expertise of specialists in cardiovascular medicine, pulmonary medicine, endovascular intervention, cardiac surgery, and radiology to identify optimal treatment pathways for patients with PE who are at increased risk for adverse outcomes.[32]

Optimal Duration of Anticoagulation
Determination of optimal duration of anticoagulation for VTE requires an assessment of the patient's long-term risk of VTE recurrence after treatment of the initial episode, as well as bleeding risk (*Figure 7*).[33] A population-based strategy recommends limited duration anticoagulation of 3-6 months for provoked VTE and indefinite duration anticoagulation for patients with low bleeding risk and unprovoked (idiopathic) VTE. Patients with malignancy and VTE comprise a population with a substantially increased risk of VTE

recurrence, and therefore are generally prescribed prolonged anticoagulation as long as their cancer is active. Warfarin[33] and the NOACs[17,34,35] have also been shown to be safe and effective for long-term prevention of recurrent VTE in patients with an unprovoked (idiopathic) event.

Aspirin may also play a role in the prevention of recurrence in patients with unprovoked VTE who may not be long-term anticoagulation candidates or who are unwilling to take an anticoagulant for an extended duration.[36]

Key Points

- NOACs are safe and effective and facilitate oral anticoagulation, compared with warfarin, in patients with VTE.

- Determination of optimal duration of anticoagulation for VTE requires an assessment of the patient's long-term risk of VTE recurrence after treatment of the initial episode and bleeding risk.

Prevention of Venous Thromboembolism

Although the use of VTE prophylaxis should be virtually universal among hospitalized patients, implementation of both mechanical and pharmacological prophylactic measures continues to be inconsistent worldwide.[37] Accordingly, the incidence of VTE among hospitalized patients, especially on medical services, remains unacceptably high.

Prophylactic Modalities
Mechanical prophylactic measures, including graduated compression stockings and intermittent pneumatic compression devices, should be considered in at-risk patients who are not candidates for pharmacological thromboprophylaxis. Pharmacological agents are recommended as first-line for prevention of VTE and include warfarin, rivaroxaban, aspirin, and subcutaneously administered UFH, LMWH, and fondaparinux, with specific recommendations varying by patient population.

Duration of Prophylaxis
The risk of VTE persists after hospital discharge in a substantial proportion of patients. Extended pharmacological VTE prophylaxis for up to 4-6 weeks in high-risk patient populations, such as those undergoing oncologic or orthopedic surgery, has been validated. Extended duration thromboprophylaxis to prevent VTE after hospital discharge in medical patients has not been proven to provide a net benefit.

Key Point

- Prevention of VTE is a crucial component of the care of hospitalized patients.

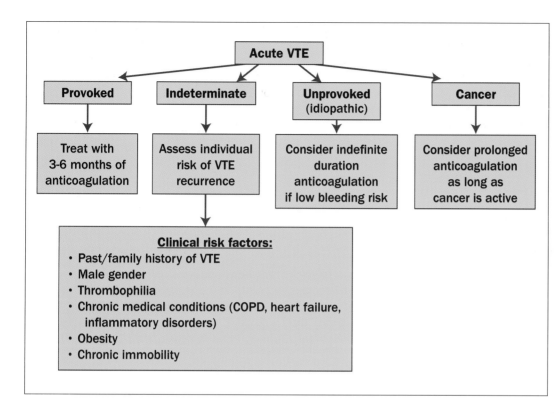

Figure 7

An Approach to Optimizing Duration of Anticoagulation in Patients With VTE

COPD = chronic obstructive pulmonary disease;
VTE = venous thromboembolism.

Long-Term Sequelae of Venous Thromboembolism

Long-term sequelae of DVT and PE contribute to the increased morbidity and mortality associated with VTE. Post-thrombotic syndrome may complicate DVT and describes a spectrum of findings ranging from chronic lower extremity discomfort and edema to venous ulceration.[1]

Chronic thromboembolic pulmonary hypertension may follow both single and recurrent episodes of PE and is characterized by persistent macrovascular obstruction, vasoconstriction, and a secondary small-vessel arteriopathy.[2] While many patients are initially asymptomatic, chronic thromboembolic pulmonary hypertension frequently presents as exercise intolerance and chronic dyspnea and may culminate in RV failure.

Pulmonary thromboendarterectomy is the most effective therapy for chronic thromboembolic pulmonary hypertension in anatomically appropriate candidates with proximal disease. Advanced medical therapy, including pulmonary vasodilators, may be considered in patients with inoperable disease or those with persistent or recurrent pulmonary hypertension after pulmonary thromboendarterectomy.

Future Directions

Future areas of research include exploring the epidemiological association and pathophysiological link between inflammation and VTE.[7] In addition, the impact of the NOACs on VTE treatment and prevention remains to be defined further in specific populations, such as those with malignancy. The safety and efficacy of emerging techniques in advanced therapy for high-risk PE and DVT, such as catheter-based "pharmacomechanical" therapy, warrant further evaluation in the clinical trial setting.

Suggested Reading

1. Agnelli G, Becattini C. Acute pulmonary embolism. N Engl J Med 2010;363:266-74.

References

1. Kahn SR, Comerota AJ, Cushman M, et al. The postthrombotic syndrome: evidence-based prevention, diagnosis, and treatment strategies: a scientific statement from the American Heart Association. Circulation 2014;130:1636-61.

2. Piazza G, Goldhaber SZ. Chronic thromboembolic pulmonary hypertension. N Engl J Med 2011;364:351-60.

3. Huang W, Goldberg RJ, Anderson FA, Kiefe CI, Spencer FA. Secular trends in occurrence of acute venous thromboembolism: the Worcester VTE study (1985-2009). Am J Med 2014;127:829-39.e5.

4. Park B, Messina L, Dargon P, Huang W, Ciocca R, Anderson FA. Recent trends in clinical outcomes and resource utilization for pulmonary embolism in the United States: findings from the nationwide inpatient sample. Chest 2009;136:983-90.

5. Sogaard KK, Schmidt M, Pedersen L, Horvath-Puho E, Sorensen HT. 30-year mortality after venous thromboembolism: a population-based cohort study. Circulation 2014;130:829-36.

6. Piazza G. Thrombophilia testing, recurrent thrombosis, and women's health. Circulation 2014;130:283-7.

7. Piazza G. Beyond Virchow's Triad: does cardiovascular inflammation explain the recurrent nature of venous thromboembolism? Vasc Med 2015;20:102-4.

8. Folsom AR, Lutsey PL, Astor BC, Cushman M. C-reactive protein and venous thromboembolism. A prospective investigation in the ARIC cohort. Thromb Haemost 2009;102:615-9.

9. Glynn RJ, Danielson E, Fonseca FA, et al. A randomized trial of rosuvastatin in the prevention of venous thromboembolism. N Engl J Med 2009;360:1851-61.

10. Piazza G. Submassive pulmonary embolism. JAMA 2013;309:171-80.

11. Trujillo-Santos J, den Exter PL, Gomez V, et al. Computed tomography-assessed right ventricular dysfunction and risk stratification of patients with acute non-massive pulmonary embolism: systematic review and meta-analysis. J Thromb Haemost 2013;11:1823-32.

12. Piazza G. Venous thromboembolism and cancer. Circulation 2013;128:2614-8.

13. Kimmel SE, French B, Kasner SE, et al. A pharmacogenetic versus a clinical algorithm for warfarin dosing. N Engl J Med 2013;369:2283-93.

14. Pirmohamed M, Burnside G, Eriksson N, et al. A randomized trial of genotype-guided dosing of warfarin. N Engl J Med 2013;369:2294-303.

15. Verhoef TI, Ragia G, de Boer A, et al. A randomized trial of genotype-guided dosing of acenocoumarol and phenprocoumon. N Engl J Med 2013;369:2304-12.

16. Agnelli G, Buller HR, Cohen A, et al. Oral apixaban for the treatment of acute venous thromboembolism. N Engl J Med 2013;369:799-808.

17. Bauersachs R, Berkowitz SD, Brenner B, et al. Oral rivaroxaban for symptomatic venous thromboembolism. N Engl J Med 2010;363:2499-510.

18. Buller HR, Decousus H, Grosso MA, et al. Edoxaban versus warfarin for the treatment of symptomatic venous thromboembolism. N Engl J Med 2013;369:1406-15.

19. Buller HR, Prins MH, Lensin AW, et al. Oral rivaroxaban for the treatment of symptomatic pulmonary embolism. N Engl J Med 2012;366:1287-97.

20. Schulman S, Kakkar AK, Goldhaber SZ, et al. Treatment of acute venous thromboembolism with dabigatran or warfarin and pooled analysis. Circulation 2014;129:764-72.

21. Schulman S, Kearon C, Kakkar AK, et al. Dabigatran versus warfarin in the treatment of acute venous thromboembolism. N Engl J Med 2009;361:2342-52.

22. Jaff MR, McMurtry MS, Archer SL, et al. Management of massive and submassive pulmonary embolism, iliofemoral deep vein thrombosis, and chronic thromboembolic pulmonary hypertension: a scientific statement from the American Heart Association. Circulation 2011;123:1788-830.

23. Kearon C, Akl EA, Comerota AJ, et al. Antithrombotic therapy for VTE disease: Antithrombotic Therapy and Prevention of Thrombosis, 9th ed: American College of Chest Physicians Evidence-Based Clinical Practice Guidelines. Chest 2012;141:e419S-94S.

24. Konstantinides SV, Torbicki A, Agnelli G, et al. 2014 ESC Guidelines on the diagnosis and management of acute pulmonary embolism. Eur Heart J 2014;35:3033-69.

25. Meyer G, Vicaut E, Danays T, et al. Fibrinolysis for patients with intermediate-risk pulmonary embolism. N Engl J Med 2014;370:1402-11.

26. Chatterjee S, Chakraborty A, Weinberg I, et al. Thrombolysis for pulmonary embolism and risk of all-cause mortality, major bleeding, and intracranial hemorrhage: a meta-analysis. JAMA 2014;311:2414-21.

27. Marti C, John G, Konstantinides S, et al. Systemic thrombolytic therapy for acute pulmonary embolism: a systematic review and meta-analysis. Eur Heart J 2015;36:605-14.

28. Kucher N, Boekstegers P, Muller O, et al. Randomized controlled trial of ultrasound-assisted catheter-directed thrombolysis for acute intermediate-risk pulmonary embolism. Circulation 2014;129:479-86.

29. Piazza G, Hohlfelder B, Jaff MR, et al. A prospective, single-arm, multicenter trial of ultrasound-facilitated catheter-directed low-dose fibrinolysis for acute massive and submassive pulmonary embolism (SEATTLE II) 2014. Presented on March 30, 2014, at the American College of Cardiology Annual Scientific Session, Washington, DC.

30. Poterucha TJ, Bergmark B, Aranki S, Kaneko T, Piazza G. Surgical pulmonary embolectomy. Circulation 2015;132:1146-51.

31. Mismetti P, Laporte S, Pellerin O, et al. Effect of a retrievable inferior vena cava filter plus anticoagulation vs anticoagulation alone on risk of recurrent pulmonary embolism: a randomized clinical trial. JAMA 2015;313:1627-35.

32. Dudzinski DM, Piazza G. Multidisciplinary pulmonary embolism response teams. Circulation 2016;133:98-103.

33. Goldhaber SZ, Piazza G. Optimal duration of anticoagulation after venous thromboembolism. Circulation 2011;123:664-7.

34. Agnelli G, Buller HR, Cohen A, et al. Apixaban for extended treatment of venous thromboembolism. N Engl J Med 2013;368:699-708.

35. Schulman S, Kearon C, Kakkar AK, et al. Extended use of dabigatran, warfarin, or placebo in venous thromboembolism. N Engl J Med 2013;368:709-18.

36. Simes J, Becattini C, Agnelli G, et al., on behalf of INSPIRE Study Investigators (International Collaboration of Aspirin Trials for Recurrent Venous Thromboembolism). Aspirin for the prevention of recurrent venous thromboembolism: the INSPIRE collaboration. Circulation 2014;130:1062-71.

37. Cohen AT, Tapson VF, Bergmann JF, et al., on behalf of ENDORSE Investigators. Venous thromboembolism risk and prophylaxis in the acute hospital care setting (ENDORSE study): a multinational cross-sectional study. Lancet 2008;371:387-94.